Fundamental Aspects of Legal, Ethical and Professional Issues in Nursing

Maggie Reeves and Jacquie Orford

Quay
Books

Mark Allen
Publishing Ltd

Quay Books Division, Mark Allen Publishing Limited, Jesses Farm,
Snow Hill, Dinton, Salisbury, Wiltshire SP3 5HN

British Library Cataloguing-in-Publication Data
A catalogue record is available for this book

© Mark Allen Publishing Limited 2002
ISBN 1 85642 209 7

Printed in the UK by Bath Press, Bath

Contents

Acknowledgements

We would like to acknowledge the help of the many people who have assisted in the writing of this book.

Firstly, we thank the many students and colleagues with whom we have worked during our nursing and teaching careers. During this time we have learnt how to answer questions and to find out answers, and to try to give these answers at the level the individual could understand. Students, in particular, have tested us to ensure that they have got the answer to their satisfaction and have challenged us with examples from clinical practice — some of which are included in this book. Without this learning, this book could not have been written.

Secondly, we thank those who have offered advice and information over the years and have contributed to our knowledge levels. Special thanks go to Mary Meynell, a former colleague who set the scene for many of our legal, ethical and professional teaching sessions. Our specific thanks go to George Castledine and Bridgit Dimond for reading through the manuscript, and all the other authors acknowledged through the text.

Our final thanks go to Mike Reeves and Steve, Christopher and Victoria Orford for 'putting up with' our book writing, and the inconvenience this often causes.

We would like to dedicate this book to students past and present and hope that the *Fundamental Aspects of Legal, Ethical and Professional Issues in Nursing* will be a helpful tool for study and in nursing practice.

Maggie Reeves
Jacquie Orford
April 2002

Foreword

We are going through a time of considerable change in the health service in this country, and there is an urgent need for all nurses to understand the professional implications of this. Some of the key issues emerging are of course closely linked to the National Health Service Plan, and the proposals for the future regulation of the healthcare professions.

The United Kingdom Central Council for Nursing, Midwifery and Health Visiting (UKCC), and the National Nursing Boards have disappeared and in their place is a new organisation with a new purpose and new ideas. Greater public involvement is starting to put the health professions under more scrutiny and pressure for improved quality in areas such as ethical and professional decision making and participation in services.

The Nursing and Midwifery Council (NMC) has taken over the future of regulation of nurses and midwives and is now the new body which is determined to reaffirm established standards and guidelines and to develop new ones.

Every nurse should not only be able to demonstrate that they have an awareness of the legislation and policy which is providing the future framework within which health care is delivered, but also that they should have a good grasp of the fundamental legal, ethical and professional aspects which are involved.

In order to accomplish this in the limited time often available for studying and keeping up-to-date, there is a need for both relevant and pertinent information to be easily available and accessible for nurses, as well as being presented clearly, concisely and precisely.

This excellent little book by Maggie Reeves and Jacquie Orford, sets out to accomplish an ideal introduction to the subject, and after reading through it, I am sure that you will be as convinced as I am that it achieves its aims.

Students on pre-registration nursing programmes will find this an essential book to guide them in their understanding of such issues as accountability, liability, truthfulness, truth-telling, choice, consent, autonomy, and advocacy.

The book starts simply and develops into a well-balanced and detailed account of the professional implications of some of the most important issues for nurses.

This makes the book applicable for all students of nursing, and a very handy reference for all registered nurses, especially those working in clinical practice.

There are various suggestions sprinkled throughout the book relating to activities to help the reader reflect on the subject matter and the use of a special symbol to help bring this together.

The final part of the book covers the principles of written communication and each section is well supported by references and essential reading.

It has given me great pleasure to read through this text and I can strongly recommend it to all those nurses who want not only a simple and straightforward approach to the subject, but a quick and easy reference.

George Castledine, July 2002
Professor and Consultant of General Nursing,
University of Central England, Birmingham,
and Dudley Group of Hospitals NHS Trust

Introduction

This book is aimed at those who are new to the fundamental concepts of legal, ethical and professional issues in nursing and may want help in understanding them. This may be student nurses whenever they are introduced to these themes in their pre-registration nursing programme or for qualified nurses who are supervising such students in clinical practice.

Many people find the more advanced books on these subjects difficult to follow and want something to provide a foundation for them. Hopefully, this book will do this.

It will look at the three issues in nursing — legal, professional and ethical — as separate entities. This is to help the reader understand these concepts in a better way. Although these topics will be looked at separately, in clinical nursing practice they are nearly always combined together. One way of imagining this is to consider a plait of hair. Each of the three strands is separate, but when plaited the woven hair is one.

When this occurs in the book you will see this symbol to guide you.

The law and ethics are the framework in which professional issues are discussed and measured. This does not mean that the law has no morals or there is no law in professional aspects of nursing. The plait is used as a visual tool.

The Health Service Circular 219.99 (Department of Health [DoH], 1999) introduced the requirements for a revised nursing education programme. The specific learning outcomes for this programme were devised by the United Kingdom Central Council for Nursing, Midwifery and Health Visiting (UKCC, 2001a). This book will help students successfully achieve the following UKCC's learning outcomes.

Outcomes to be achieved for entry to the branch programme

❖ Discuss in an informed manner the implications of professional regulation for nursing practice.

❖ Demonstrate an awareness of the UKCC's *Code of professional conduct*.

❖ Demonstrate an awareness of, and apply ethical principles to, nursing practice.

❖ Demonstrate an awareness of legislation relevant to nursing practice.

❖ Demonstrate the importance of promoting equity in patient and client care by contributing to nursing care in a fair and anti-discriminatory way.

❖ Contribute to the development and documentation... about (*sic*) the needs of patients and clients.

❖ Contribute... involving patients and clients... helping patients and clients to make informed decisions.

❖ Demonstrate responsibility for one's own learning through the development of a portfolio of practice and recognise when further learning is required.

Competencies for entry to the register

❖ Manage oneself, one's practice, and that of others, in accordance with the UKCC's *Code of professional conduct*, recognising one's own abilities and limitations.

❖ Practise in accordance with an ethical and legal framework which ensures the primacy of patient and client interest and well being and respects confidentiality.

❖ Practise in a fair and anti-discriminatory way, acknowledging the differences in beliefs and cultural practices of individuals or groups.

❖ Formulate and document... where possible in partnership with patients, clients, their carers and family and friends, within a framework of informed consent.

❖ Provide a rationale for the nursing care delivered which takes account of social, cultural, spiritual, legal, political and economic influences.

❖ Demonstrate key skills.

❖ Demonstrate a commitment to the need for continuing professional development and personal supervision activities in order to enhance knowledge, skills, values and attitudes needed for safe and effective nursing practice.

The authors are fully aware that this book has been published at the same time as the Nursing and Midwifery Council (NMC) has come into being. Sometimes it will seem confusing to refer to both the UKCC and the NMC but this is essential to understand the changing professional climate.

The reader will be invited to cross reference the subjects in this book with all the learning outcomes (UKCC, 2001a) and also the UKCC's and NMC's *Code of professional conduct* (UKCC, 1992a; NMC, 2002), the latter reference being the new edition of the *Code of professional conduct* (see *Appendix 1*). This new document is a combination and update of the UKCC's (1992a) *Code of professional conduct, Scope of Professional Practice* (UKCC, 1992b) and *Guidelines for professional practice* (UKCC, 1996). It is hoped that by doing this the book will be much more useful.

To get the most out of this book we suggest that you have a dedicated notebook/file which you will use to undertake the recommended activities to enhance your learning and reflection. This work can then be incorporated into your personal professional profile (UKCC, 2001b). This, in turn, will help you to maintain and improve your professional knowledge and competence (UKCC, 1992a: Clause 3; NMC, 2002: Clause 6).

All references can be found in the chapter reference lists except:

Department of Health (1999) Health Service Circular HSC 1999/219 *Making a Difference: Strengthening the nursing, midwifery and health visiting contribution to health and health care*. DoH, London

United Kingdom Central Council for Nursing, Midwifery and Health Visiting (1992b) *Scope of Professional Practice*. UKCC, London

Section I

To open this section there are some important words and definitions to introduce.

> ❖ **Legal** will be looking at different aspects of the **law**.
> ❖ **Professional** will be looking at how nurses behave and perform in **practice**.
> ❖ **Ethical** will be looking at different issues related to **conscience**.

Although these topics will be looked at separately, in clinical nursing practice they are nearly always combined together. One way of imagining this is to consider a plait of hair. Each of the three strands is separate, but when plaited the woven hair is one. The law and ethics are the framework in which professional issues are discussed and measured.

What is law?

The aim of this first part of *Section 1* is to ensure that you have a basic understanding of the origin of law and its relevance to your nursing practice. It will cover aspects such as the main categories of law and how they are created. You will be given the opportunity to begin to identify some specific laws which influence nursing and health care.

The term liability will be defined, criminal and civil liability will be briefly explained and some comparisons made between the two. Some offences that the nurse could commit will be identified. The court system will be discussed so that you can gain an appreciation of the process in which you or a patient/client may become involved.

A broad understanding of the law is a requirement of many occupations today and the general public is increasingly becoming aware of their rights in law. Health care and nursing are no exception. The new *Code of professional conduct* states that registered nurses and midwives must also adhere to the laws of the country in which they are practising (NMC, 2002; *Appendix 1*).

Student nurses who are undertaking pre-registration education programmes also have to abide by the standards set by the UKCC and NMC for registered nurses, midwives and health visitors, although they practice under supervision. One of the UKCC's learning outcomes which student nurses need to achieve by the end of their first year requires that they, 'demonstrate an awareness of legislation relevant to nursing practice' (UKCC, 2001a). This achievement is required in both theory and practice.

Where does law in the United Kingdom come from?

For simplicity, the focus will be on England and Wales which share the primary legislation of Westminster, but you need to be aware that there are many similarities with Scotland and Northern Ireland. There are also some differences and, as a result of new legislation in 1998, Scotland and Northern Ireland can now make some laws relevant to their own country. This includes those relating to health issues (Elliott and Quinn, 2000).

There are two main origins of law, one made through Parliament (statutory law), the other from case law (common law). There are also laws which are affected by laws laid down in Europe.

1. **Statutory law** has been laid down and passed through Parliament and is often referred to as being on the statute book. It is known as an Act of Parliament and is given a specific title and a date when it has completed the necessary stages.
2. **Common law** has evolved over a considerable period of time and is based upon cases which have set a precedent. The judgements made are often referred to in subsequent cases and act as a 'yardstick' against which future decisions are made. One of the purposes of this is to try and ensure equity in decision-making. Common law can be traced back in some instances to twelfth and thirteenth century England, although the punishments given out today are very different from those meted out in the Middle Ages!

How is statutory law created through Parliament?

There are a series of stages that are followed in both the House of Commons and the House of Lords but they occur at different time intervals. A proposed piece of law may be first introduced in the House of Commons as a Bill. A Member of Parliament (MP), who is often a member of the government of the time introduces it. There are also Private Members' Bills. These are proposed by backbench MPs who have an interest in a particular subject which they believe should become law. An example is the **Medical Treatment (Prevention of Euthanasia) Bill** presented by Ann Winterton, MP in 1999 which failed to become law due to deep concerns expressed by the Government who did not support the bill (Royal College of Nursing [RCN], 2000). Some Bills may be first introduced in the House of Lords.

Usually a **green paper** is published which is distributed for consultation to interested parties such as national health service trusts or health professional bodies if the topic is health related. The green paper is often amended as a result of suggestions from a variety of sources including pressure groups, or even an individual who can be quite influential.

A **white paper** follows, setting out what the Government intends to do. The subsequent bill goes through a series of readings and stages (*Figure 1.1*), starting by giving it a title followed by an outline of the general principles (second reading). Voting takes place and a majority is needed for progression to the next stage. Once the general principles have been presented a committee is formed which develop these in much more detail.

The committee is important because it produces a detailed report for further consideration.

At the **report stage**, which is debated before the full House of Commons, amendments can be made. Voting occurs and if successful the process of the three readings occurs in the House of Lords.

Eventually, if both houses are in agreement with all the amendments the bill goes to the Monarch for **Royal Assent**; this signature transforming it to an Act of Parliament. However, the Act does not necessarily come into force (ie. become law) when the monarch signs it. Dates are set either in the Act itself or fixed by 'Statutory Instruments'. Interestingly, some Acts have never been brought into force.

This process can be very slow, complex and time-consuming

and the bill may just run out of time, never to become law. There is also a variety of delaying tactics which can be employed to exacerbate the situation.

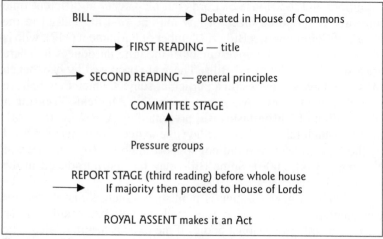

Figure 1.1: The process of creating statutory law

Activity: Make a list of at least five Acts of Parliament which you think are relevant to nursing. Try to include the date that the Act was passed.

There are a vast number of Acts which affect nursing and the registered nurse or student should be able to cite several by name and date. Check to see if your list contains any listed in *Figure 1.2*. The ability to discuss the key aspects and relate them to practice will ensure that the nurse does not break the law and will protect the interests of patients and clients.

Abortion Act 1967

Misuse of Drugs Act 1971

Health and Safety at Work Act 1974

Mental Health Act 1983

Public Health (Control of Diseases) Act 1984

Children Act 1989

Disability Discrimination Act 1995

Nurses, Midwives and Health Visitors Act 1997

Data Protection Act 1998

Public Interest Disclosure Act 1998

The Human Rights Act 1998

The Health Act 1999

Figure 1.2: Acts of Parliament

Some of these are under review and the interested reader may discover several amendments to the original acts. Legal texts usually contain a table of statutes if you want to check if there is an Act of Parliament about a particular issue. The important thing to remember is how these statutes affect your nursing practice.

Criminal and civil liability

> Activity: Using a dictionary find a definition of liability.
>
> You have probably come up with words such as legal obligation, being answerable for, responsible for...

A **crime** is a public wrong which is considered unacceptable to society and thus the state prosecutes the offender providing that there is sufficient evidence.

The opposite of a public wrong is a private one, whereby the offended individual (plaintiff or claimant) sues the wrongdoer in a civil action. The French word *tort* is often used in relation to these civil cases.

NB: Older texts may refer to the word 'plaintiff' but Dimond (2002) stresses that 'claimant' is the new term to be used.

> Activity: Try to compare the two types of 'wrong' and make a table of the differences.

In *Figure 1.3* the term **R** *vs* **Another** is the way a criminal case is named, whereby the **Crown Prosecution Service (CPS)** takes the case to court (**R** means Rex [King] or Regina [Queen]). **Another** is the surname of the other party involved, the accused.

In civil cases the first name (**One**) is that of the claimant while the second (**Other**) is the defendant.

The seriousness of criminal and civil cases can vary. For example, a parking offence is a minor criminal offence compared to the extremely serious wrong of negligence. To confuse the issue further, some incidents are both criminal offences and civil wrongs, eg. assault.

Criminal	Civil
Offence against the state	Civil wrong against the individual
May be intentional	Usually unintentional
Prosecuted by **CPS-R** *vs* **Another**	Sued **One** *vs* **Other**
Proof of guilt beyond all reasonable doubt	Liability on a balance of probabilities
Wide variety of sentences	
Prison, fine, community service, absolute discharge	Compensation, payment of damages, apology

Figure 1.3: Criminal *vs* civil liability

In an ideal world no nurse would ever commit a criminal offence or civil wrong but, unfortunately, some nurses do. The most serious offence would be murder. This is obviously totally unacceptable to society legally, ethically and to the profession of nursing. Murder is classed as a crime and is a common law offence and there is no such statute as a murder act.

> Activity: Using the information given so far, identify some wrongs which a nurse could commit and classify each as either criminal or civil, and either bound by statutory or common law.

Dimond (1995: 12, 23) provides some examples of definitions of certain crimes such as assault, battery, wounding and theft. She also lists some forms of civil action.

One of the most significant civil offences that may involve nurses is **negligence**, which is discussed in *Section 2, p. 41.*

Hierarchy of the Courts

There are separate criminal and civil courts in England and most cities have a variety of each. Nearly all criminal cases start out in the Magistrates Court, which is presided over by lay individuals known as Justices of the Peace (JPs). If the accused pleads guilty of a fairly minor offence it can be dealt with there. Magistrates have a limited range of sentences they can impose. In other instances the magistrate will hold committal proceedings to decide if it should go to the Crown Court.

In hierarchical order there follows County Courts and Crown Courts; Divisional Courts; High Courts; Courts of Appeal and the House of Lords in England, while beyond this are the European Courts. You may want to produce a flow chart to refer to or look at those in Dimond (1995: 6, 9), or Dimond (2002: 6, 9) for more detail.

In addition, there is the Coroner's Court which is empowered to investigate deaths which occur under specific circumstances. It functions differently from criminal and civil courts as the purpose is to find out the cause of death, not accuse anyone. Nurses may be required to attend as witnesses to answer questions if they were involved in the deceased's care.

Associated Study: You may now want to find out a little more and, apart from the activities suggested so far, you could try to follow an Act of Parliament as it is created, making a few notes in your notebook.

Valuable resources are newspapers, television and the Internet. Don't expect it to happen all at once though, remember the legislative process can be very slow!

If you have ever been called for jury service reflect on what you learned in relation to the areas covered; or follow a case as it is reported in the press or on the Internet.

Cases that have implications for nurses or health care are, of course, pertinent.

What is professional?

This second part of *Section 1* focuses on introducing professional issues.

It will start by asking you to consider the terms professional, professionalisation and professionalism. Nursing's professional bodies will be discussed and the changes that are currently taking place will be identified. You need to keep abreast of these many changes as part of your professional development. An outline of how nursing is controlled and its disciplinary procedures will be included.

The *Codes of professional conduct* (UKCC, 1992a; NMC, 2002) will be introduced and you will have an opportunity to analyse them.

The professional issues will be looked at as a separate subject and then will be woven with legal and ethical issues together with examples from nursing practice.

What does professional mean?

Many books have been written discussing the idea of profession, professional, professionalism and professionalisation. What do they all mean?

> Activity: Look up all the words in a dictionary/nursing textbooks — see reference/reading list.

You will come up with answers such as:

❖ Burnard and Chapman (1993) indicate that a **profession**:
  i) needs a body of specific knowledge based on research
  ii) has knowledge that is passed on to new entrants to a profession and is guided by members of that profession
  iii) has clients whose needs are placed before the needs of the professional

iv) recognises that accountability for standards is judged by other professionals.

The *Little Oxford Dictionary* (1986) considers that a **profession** is an occupation... especially involved in some branch of advanced learning or science.

❖ Fletcher and Buka (1999) state that a **professional** is a practitioner who has undergone a long course of training, the successful completion of which permits the candidate to be entered on to a register maintained by the ruling body of that profession... governed by statutes. The *Little Oxford Dictionary* (1986) also describes professional as the way a professional behaves — the qualities or typical features of professionals, in other words **professionalism**. Tschudin (1994) suggests that the term professionalism is not only about what a group of people are, but also what they want to be.

❖ **Professionalisation** means the process of attaining professional status. The consequence of this according to Rumbold (1999: 179) is that nurses are no longer taught that they are, nor do they see themselves as, doctors' handmaids... nurses have become independent decision makers...

Heywood Jones (1999: 93) says that graduate and diploma nursing courses have pushed nursing closer to true **professionalisation**.

It is amazing that there are so many different ways of looking at this subject. Many of the books look at the history of nursing, the process of professionalisation and the quest for professionalism. However, most will look at the nurse, midwife or health visitor as a professional and how they are expected to behave in clinical practice.

Nursing's professional bodies

The **United Kingdom Central Council for Nursing, Midwifery and Health Visiting (UKCC)** was established following the passing of the Nurses, Midwives and Health Visitors Act in 1979. There have been amendments to the 1979 Act, notably in 1992 and 1997. It is interesting to note that the professional body is concerned with the professions in its title while the legislation is named after the practitioners. Many people confuse the two when quoting from them!

Since the first Nurses, Midwives and Health Visitors Act of 1979 nursing has been regulated and controlled by the UKCC and four **National Boards**, one for each country in the United Kingdom. Several changes and developments have occurred since 1979 which have necessitated legislative amendments, culminating in a rewrite of the Act in 1997.

However these professions are never static.

The Health Act (1999) created a new body to govern nursing: the **Nursing and Midwifery Council (NMC)** which, during 2001–2002, functioned as a 'shadow body'. From spring 2002 the UKCC and National Boards ceased to exist and the NMC took over.

The members of these councils are either appointed or elected. All registered nurses, midwives and health visitors have a responsibility to be involved in the election process. The responsibility encompasses voting for candidates that the professions have nominated. This is the basis of self-regulation and it is important we take it seriously. A comparison of the UKCC and NMC structures can be found in *Appendix 2*. Although there have been changes as a result of this new body the important key functions remain.

The main purpose of the NMC is to protect the public which it does in a variety of ways, as detailed below.

Maintains a register

It maintains a register of practitioners and it controls who may or may not be listed on that register. The registration of nurses is not a recent occurrence, as it was in 1919 when nurses were first listed as having been trained to a recognised standard. The body responsible for this was the General Nursing Council, which functioned up to 1979. There was a similar body who maintained a register of midwives.

Today's register is known as a live one because it lists those who are currently practising, not those who were once nurses and are long gone. The 1992 changes to the Nurses, Midwives and Health Visitors Act opened up new parts to the register to reflect *Project 2000* pre-registration courses. A further change is planned by the NMC who are in the process of redesigning the register.

To be eligible for entry on to the register the nurse must have successfully completed a programme of training and be of suitable character, usually verified by the university or college attended.

Once on the register there are requirements that have to be fulfilled to continue practising. Renewal of registration is essential every three years (UKCC, 2001b).

Activity: What do you think is necessary for a nurse to remain on the register?

Check your views with the professional requirements below.

Answer:

❖ The nurse, midwife or health visitor must work in that capacity for a sufficient number of hours over the past five years to continue to be competent.

❖ To keep up-to-date they must demonstrate learning activities amounting to thirty-five hours in the past three years that are relevant to their practice. The learning activity can be very varied to reflect the diversity of nursing today.

❖ Each practitioner must maintain a personal professional profile/ portfolio of learning activity.

❖ Fairly obviously, the nurse must remain of good character and, as we shall see later, this means not breaking the law.

❖ Periodic re-registration requires the payment of fees every three years. Initial registration is now exempt from financial outlay.

The NMC requires that practitioners sign to verify these aspects and there is a mechanism for checking the accuracy of this.

In addition, anyone can check via the NMC that an individual's registration is current, as it is a criminal offence to claim to be a nurse when one has not qualified.

Although students are not on the register until successfully qualified, some of the requirements for renewal of registration form the basis of good practice. Students now have to keep a profile/ portfolio of their learning and must still keep within the law.

Sets standards and guidelines for education and training

The second function of the NMC is in relation to training of nurses and midwives. Institutions, health trusts and any other organisation that provides nurse education and/or practice experience have set standards which the student must meet. These are known as UKCC learning outcomes. They ensure parity throughout the UK depending on the branch of nursing the student is undertaking. For example, an awareness of legal, ethical and professional issues in relation to nursing practice are required (UKCC, 2001a). Prior to the 1992 Nurses, Midwives and Health Visitors Act it was the National Boards who provided pre-registration courses. Since then they have approved courses in institutions such as universities and colleges of nursing which train nurses. Prior to the creation of the NMC, these two activities were undertaken separately. New arrangements are now being developed by the NMC to assure the quality of pre- and post-registration education for nurses, midwives and health visitors. As health needs change so does the role of the nurse and the standards and requirements of course programmes reflect these.

The history of nursing clearly illustrates the many changes that have occurred since nurse training first began over a hundred years ago. It is a long time since nurses were apprentices learning 'on the job', following a very medically-orientated model of training culminating in a state final examination. Nurses today undertake a programme of education, use evidence and research as a basis for their practice, and are accountable to the patient, their employer, themselves, the law and the profession.

Sets standards for conduct and practice

Activity: How do you think nurses know what the standards are?

The UKCC produced and regularly updated a variety of documents for all nurses. You will be introduced to the UKCC (1992a), NMC (2002) *Codes of professional conduct* later in this section. These documents can also be used to develop local policies according to the UKCC (2001c).

All registered nurses are sent copies when they qualify and receive new versions when needed or requested. Universities may give pre-registration students these documents, particularly as the focus of the foundation component of their course is on the *Code of professional conduct.*

As the NMC website is accessible to the general public anyone can obtain a copy of any publication. This is important as it facilitates nursing's accountability to the public.

The professional bodies and practitioners regularly review these documents and feedback from the profession is an important contribution in raising standards of conduct and practice. The guidelines also form the basis upon which professional conduct is monitored.

Considers and administers procedures related to professional conduct

The NMC in its role to protect the public considers all complaints of professional misconduct. Only the key principles are discussed here, ie.

Professional conduct complaints

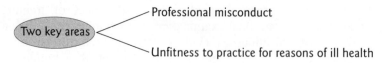

Two key areas
- Professional misconduct
- Unfitness to practice for reasons of ill health

Professional misconduct

Activity: Make a list of the types of complaint you think may be made to the professional body?

The most common complaints are about:

- ❖ Physical, sexual or verbal abuse of patients.
- ❖ Theft from patients.
- ❖ Failure to care for patients properly.
- ❖ Failure to keep proper records.
- ❖ Failure to administer medicines safely.
- ❖ Deliberately concealing unsafe practice.
- ❖ Committing serious criminal offences.

UKCC, 2000

Unfitness to practice could be a result of alcohol or drug dependency, untreated serious mental illness or a serious personality disorder.

How is a complaint made?

The procedure is set in motion once a written, signed complaint is received by the NMC stating who did what, to whom and when.

Who can make a complaint?

Anyone — patients, their relatives, visitors, colleagues from any other discipline, student nurses, managers or employers.

What happens next?

The complaint is investigated by the NMC in which evidence, statements and witnesses are gathered. This is a formalised professional procedure and the purpose is to obtain information to prove beyond reasonable doubt that there is a case to answer. The case has to be one which is serious enough to justify removing the practitioner's name from the register. Do not forget the main purpose is to protect the public, not to punish practitioners.

All complaints go to a committee formed of members of the council, practitioners and consumer representatives. Interim suspension of the nurse may occur if the offence is very serious.

Consequences:

1. Close the case.
2. Refer the complaint for a further formal hearing to the Conduct and Competence Committee.
3. Refer the complaint to the Health Committee.
4. Issue a formal caution as to future conduct which is monitored.

If the complaint is forwarded for further consideration it is heard in public to reflect the NMC's public accountability. The format of the hearing is similar to a criminal court. The aim is to determine whether the facts are proven and if this is the case, if it is serious professional misconduct. The NMC has the power to take a variety of actions depending on the outcome of the hearing.

Activity: Access the NMC website (http://www.nmc-org.uk) and identify what these actions might be.
Find out how the Health Committee may be involved, how they hear a case and the options open to them.
Make some notes in your notebook.

During 2000–2001, two hundred and twenty-one cases were sent for the full hearing to the UKCC's Professional Conduct Committee, compared to one hundred and sixty-nine cases in the previous year. For example, on 13 August, 2001 three nurses were struck off the register who had been convicted of serious offences. One related to ill treatment of a patient in a learning disabilities unit while the other two were offences committed outside work. The police referred all cases where a conviction had occurred to the UKCC so that a professional misconduct hearing could be considered. One of these offences involved the possession of 'Class A' controlled drugs outside work, and the other was trying to obtain money fraudulently from a local council by claiming housing and tax benefit while working as a nurse (UKCC, 2001d).

These examples very clearly demonstrate the profession's determination to protect the public.

All the information included about the NMC is current at the time of publication. The authors recognise that as the new organisation assumes responsibility there may be changes made to the situation described here.

This brings the discussion round to the *Code of professional conduct* (UKCC, 1992a; NMC, 2002) and the other supporting texts published by the UKCC to guide and advise nurses who must behave in an appropriate way.

Here the three strands are included yet again – legal, ethical and professional.

When the *Code of professional conduct* was written, it was constructed within the laws of England, Wales, Scotland and Northern Ireland. It was also based on ethical principles. It is therefore a **professional** document that adheres to the **law** and is able to help with **ethical** decisions.

A working knowledge of this booklet was expected by the UKCC and continues to be expected by the NMC. For the student nurse the learning outcome for entry to the branch programme is 'demonstrate an awareness of the UKCC's *Code of professional conduct*' and for entry to the register, 'practise in accordance with the UKCC's *Code of professional conduct*' (UKCC, 2001a: 10–11).

Activity: To summarise the 'professional section', answer the following questions. Most of the answers can be found in this text, using your own knowledge and also using the reading highlighted at the end of this section.

* If the *Code of professional conduct* is a guide or a standard, what purpose does it serve?
* Who is it designed for?
* Who wrote it?
* Name the law that established the body that wrote it?
* How many clauses does it contain?
* What types of issues are covered in the clauses?
* What power does it have?
* What consequences could arise from putting the code into practice or ignoring its content?

What is ethics?

Ethics is a subject used every day. You may not identify any decisions made as using 'ethics' but whatever you do in life there are reasons why you follow certain paths.

People over the centuries have looked at why individuals follow different paths and have considered frameworks to identify trends. This is loosely what ethical theory is.

Thompson *et al* (2000) define ethics (which is from the Greek word 'ethos' — the spirit of a community) as the collective belief-and-value system of any moral community, social or professional group. It is one of the ways by which a group/community can live in harmony.

This definition introduces two more words that require definition: 'morals' and 'values'.

Again according to Thompson *et al* (2000), morals and morality (from the Latin word 'mores') refer to the domain of personal values and rules of behaviour and rules of conduct regulating social interactions.

Morality and ethics deal with human relationships — how humans treat other beings so as to promote mutual welfare, growth, creativity and meaning as they strive for good over bad and right over wrong (Thiroux, 2001).

A value is very personal and is, according to Simon (1973),

> *One of a set of personal beliefs and attitudes about the truth, beauty and worth of any thought, object or behaviour. Values are action oriented and give direction and meaning to one's life.*

They are the starting points for morality and ethics.

These three concepts of values, morals and ethics can be seen to interact and relate to each other in an individual quite comfortably. Each person's morals and ethics develop during a lifetime and originate from a variety of things valued. Thus, these values and morals have been acquired from a variety of sources, which will be looked at in this section.

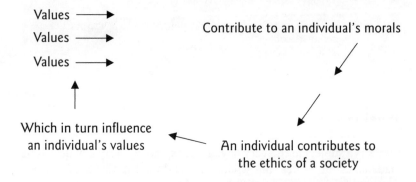

These concepts and definitions will now be pulled together to make more sense of them.

What is a value?

What is a value?

Activity: Try to think of another definition of a value, and then consider what you value and why.

Not an easy thing to do!

Perhaps your definition of a value indicated that it was something that is very important to you, it is personal, precious and very often it is something that you would take risks to defend.

Burnard and Chapman (1993) suggest that to find out what a person values and why it is valued, it would be useful to look at anthropology, geography, sociology, psychology and theology as related to that individual. How do all these 'ologies' help you decide who or what has influenced what you value?

Activity: Consider all the 'ologies' listed above and relate them to your personal circumstances.

Possible answers which also raise further questions:

❖ Looking at 'anthropology' could identify your cultural background and your social situation.

  Where were you brought up?
  What was expected of you as a child in different circumstances?
  What sort of family you were raised in?
  Apart from your family, who else had influence over you in your childhood?

❖ 'Geography' may identify the environment that you have been brought up in and exposed to.

What are your attitudes towards conservation, smoking, urban areas, animals, rural areas, beggars, water and sunlight?

❖ 'Sociology' may help you analyse 'why' you value certain things and the influence those around you had (have?) on you.

Who has influenced you the most throughout your life — a person(s) or a group of people?
Do you still value the things that the person(s) mentioned above value(d)?
If you no longer value these things, why?

❖ 'Psychology' on the other hand may indicate what sort of person you are and why you respond to external influences as you do.

Are you easily persuaded to change your mind?
Are you aware of how you tend to respond to different circumstances?
Do you find advertising easily or rarely influences you?

❖ 'Theology' may also be a great influence on your value system and be tied up with the other issues looked at above. Your spiritual or religious point of view may be the most significant factor of all.

When you make a decision does your religious (or otherwise) belief system influence what you do?
Do you find you value things which others seem to consider unimportant?
Are you conscious of 'trying to do the right thing'?
Are your beliefs about 'right' and 'wrong' different from some of your colleagues?

Taking all your answers to the above questions you may have begun to start thinking about what you actually value and where you first got that notion.

Activity: Here are some other things for you to consider:

❖ Look at each section and decide what it is you actually value — make a list.
❖ Now take your list and put your most important value at the top and then prioritise the rest.
❖ Look back several years and ask yourself if each one was a value then and whether it was as important to you.

Tschudin (1992) argues that values are not static, they are like the rudder of our lives... and they can also be the means and instruments for making decisions, be ends in themselves and define us as persons. Values can be seen as dynamic in that they change and develop throughout life. Not all values are held to be as important as others. There is a tendency to put them into hierarchies.

An hierarchy is where something is at the top of your priorities and other values are of lesser importance. There will be some things on your list that you will never change. They are fundamentally 'you'. Within the *Code of professional conduct* (UKCC, 1992a: Clause 8; NMC, 2002: Clause 2.3) there is reference to 'conscientious objection'. This concept relates to an issue contrary to your moral beliefs, a strongly held value such as the sanctity of life, which you are never prepared to compromise. However, other things will be more flexible and adaptable.

For example: do you value your health? Very few people would say 'no' to that question. How do you value your health could be a more searching question. The following are some of the answers that student nurses have given:

- taking care when crossing the road
- keeping fit
- eating a healthy diet
- visiting the dentist regularly and keeping teeth clean
- practising safe sex
- trying to keep stress free.

Look at one of these answers to see how it could be adapted.

Many people aim at eating a healthy diet. Those who truly eat a healthy diet may on occasions eat very unhealthily. This does not mean that they do not value a healthy diet, but that the individual can be flexible about this particular value.

Another value such as the sanctity of life may be more difficult to compromise. This could be an individual's bedrock value that will never change despite circumstances.

One of the important things about looking at values is that you clarify for yourself what concepts you value. This clarification can help you understand why from a negative point of view another nurse or a patient irritates you so much. The nurse, for example, may value the concept of 'work' in a different way; the patient because his manners are culturally different from yours. Conversely, your friends may all have the same approach to the balance of academic work and social life. People often make friends with those who share similar values.

This section has been quite detailed because as Uustal (1978) warned, 'if you do not take time to examine and articulate your values, you will not be fully effective with patients'. This could also relate to your personal relationships as well.

What you value influences your moral behaviour and the decisions that you make in life. Your values can also be the frameworks on which you judge others. It is important to remember this when considering the often repeated phrase — nurses must be non-judgemental. Perhaps it is wise to acknowledge that we do judge others but remember that this judgement must not affect the way we nurse. It is what we do with our judgements rather than having them in the first place. This is when a nurse (midwife or health visitor) behaves in a professional manner.

Now refer back to the diagram and see that although you may have many and varied values, they all contribute to your personal set of morals. Each person has a different set depending on all the 'ologies' referred to earlier. Your life experiences may also have affected how you react to your past values and those of others. Individually, however, our consciences are sensitive to these values. These values may make you aware of factors that prick your conscience and help you decide the appropriate path.

> Activity: Because people are all different, the things that affect your conscience may be different from your friend's. Consider:
>
> ❖ What affects your conscience?
> ❖ What helps you decide what is right or wrong?
> ❖ What feelings do you experience/what reactions do you receive if you do, i) right or ii) wrong?
> ❖ What do you do if someone else takes a different approach from you?

The answers you have given will be very personal, but there will be words that are common to all. Statements like 'feeling guilty', 'feeling uncomfortable with myself', 'angry with myself' and 'worried about what others think' have all been expressed by students in the past. Equally, there are reactions when something 'right' has been done, feelings of smugness, relief or regret. Other people may not appreciate you 'doing the right thing' because it in turn makes them feel guilty. Their reaction may be one of hostility, rejection or hurt.

Such reactions could lead to a confrontation or being ignored. Acceptance of another's viewpoint is not a straightforward thing. If you value something you will defend it and so will the other person!

Relating values and morals to nursing practice

In nursing, as in life in general, you are presented with all sorts of situations to which you will react. Problems come to you that have to be dealt with. The way you deal with each problem will be based on the values that you have and the moral standpoint that you take.

Many of the problems you face have to do with things like honesty, doing good, having a choice, valuing someone's worth and being fair about something.

Philosophers have tried to put these issues into a coherent order. Thiroux (2001) is one such philosopher who has made quite a simple list of ideas into which values could slot. His list/framework or set of principles provides a way of looking at such issues. They could be quite minor in character or be very weighty issues indeed.

His list consists of the following:

The value of life: he suggests that individuals should revere life and accept death.

Goodness or rightness: to promote goodness over badness (sometimes called beneficence), to cause no harm or badness (sometimes called non-maleficence), to prevent badness or harm.

Justice or fairness: equality of distribution.

Honesty or truth-telling: providing meaningful communication.

Individual freedom or autonomy: freedom of individuals with individual differences to choose their own ways and means of being moral — within the framework of the above four principles.

Activity: Consider each of the following principles and scenarios. Work on each scenario and accompanying questions. You could work on your own or discuss the issues raised with friends.

Further examples are debated in Castledine (2002).

The value of life

Two qualified nurses were brought before the UKCC's Professional Conduct Committee. One of their patients with severe learning disabilities would eat her food, regurgitate it and then re-feed herself.

After a meal this client was placed on the toilet and tied to it (to prevent her falling). The two nurses then went for their meal break.

One hour later a healthcare assistant found this patient dead from aspiration of stomach contents.

> ❖ Discuss the value of life principle in this situation.
> ❖ Consider any literature you may find.
> ❖ Discuss what alternative courses of action the practitioners could have taken to prevent a similar situation.
> ❖ Which Clause(s) of the *Code of professional conduct* (NMC, 2002) is/are relevant in this scenario?

Goodness or Rightness

A visitor to the ward states that he is a senior community liaison nurse (without an ID badge) and wants to see a patient's notes prior to sorting out discharge requirements with the patient.

> ❖ Discuss the principle of goodness or rightness in this situation.
> ❖ Consider any literature you may find.
> ❖ Debate alternative strategies you might employ if you were approached by this visitor and the consequences of each.
> ❖ Which Clause(s) of the *Code of professional conduct* (NMC, 2002) is/are relevant in this scenario?

Justice or fairness

Nurses are very often short of time. Your ward is very busy and one of your student colleagues is admitted to your ward. You spend ages talking to her. Another patient (an awkward, ungrateful and rather smelly lady) is really lonely and asks you to listen to something. You say you are sorry, but you are too busy.

> ❖ Discuss the principle of justice or fairness in this situation.
> ❖ Consider any literature you may find — do not forget other UKCC booklets.
> ❖ Debate your reasons for giving preference to one patient and the consequences of this.
> ❖ Which Clause(s) of the *Code of professional conduct* (NMC, 2002) is/are relevant in this scenario?

Truth-telling or honesty

A male patient who is married with a young child is diagnosed as HIV positive. You know from discussions with him that he has other sexual partners. His wife asks you what is wrong with her husband.

> ❖ Discuss the principle of truth-telling or honesty in this situation.
> ❖ Consider any literature you may find.
> ❖ Debate alternative strategies you might employ if asked this question and the consequences of each.
> ❖ Which Clause(s) of the *Code of professional conduct* (NMC, 2002) is/are relevant in this scenario?

Individual freedom or autonomy

For several days a seventeen-year-old patient has refused to eat and drink. When you ask her why, she says it is because of her religious principles.

> ❖ Discuss the principle of individual freedom or autonomy in this situation.
> ❖ Consider any literature you may find.
> ❖ Debate the different reactions from people involved in the life of this teenager, and the potential consequences of her decision.
> ❖ Which Clause(s) of the *Code of professional conduct* (NMC, 2002) is/are relevant in this scenario?

You will notice from the questions asked following each scenario that the *Code of professional conduct* has been referred to on each occasion. This was a deliberate ploy!

 The questions may begin to illustrate the 'plait' referred to earlier. Although legal, ethical and professional issues are separate, in nursing practice they are normally entwined.

References

Burnard P, Chapman CM (1993) *Professional & Ethical Issues in Nursing: The Code of professional conduct.* 2nd edn. Baillière Tindall, London

Castledine G (2002) *Nurses Behaving Badly.* Quay Books, Mark Allen Publishing Ltd, Salisbury, Wiltshire

Chadwick R, Tadd W (1992) *Ethics & Nursing Practice. A Case Study Approach.* Macmillan, London

Dimond B (1995) *Legal Aspects of Nursing.* 2nd edn. Prentice Hall, London

Dimond B (2002) *Legal Aspects of Nursing.* 3rd edn. Longman, Harlow

Elliott C, Quinn F (2000) *English Legal System.* 3rd edn. Longman, Harlow

Fletcher L, Buka P (1999) *A Legal Framework for Caring.* Macmillan, Basingstoke

Heywood Jones I, ed. (1999) *The UKCC Code of conduct — a critical guide.* Nursing Times Books, London

Hunt G, ed. (1994) *Ethical Issues in Nursing.* Routledge, London

Nursing and Midwifery Council (2002) *Code of professional conduct.* NMC, London

Royal College of Nursing (2000) *Ethics Bulletin.* Spring edn. RCN, London

Rumbold G (1999) *Ethics in Nursing Practice.* 3rd edn. Baillière Tindall, London

Simon SB (1973) Meeting yourself halfway. Cited in: Tschudin V (1992) *Values, A Primer for Nurses.* Baillière Tindall, London

Thompson IE, Melia KM, Boyd KM (2000) *Nursing Ethics.* 4th edn. Churchill Livingstone, Edinburgh

Thiroux JP (2001) *Ethics: Theory & Practice.* 7th edn. Prentice Hall, New Jersey

Tschudin V (1994) *Deciding Ethically.* Baillière Tindall, London

Uustal D (1978) Values clarification in nursing: Application to practice. *Am J Nurs* Dec: 2053–63

United Kingdom Central Council for Nursing, Midwifery and Health Visiting (1992a) *Code of professional conduct.* 3rd edn. UKCC. London

United Kingdom Central Council for Nursing, Midwifery and Health Visiting (2000) *Complaints about professional misconduct.* UKCC, London: last updated November 2001, accessed 12.12.01 http://www.ukcc.org.uk/compc

United Kingdom Central Council for Nursing, Midwifery and Health Visiting (2001a) *Requirements for pre-registration nursing programmes.* UKCC, London

United Kingdom Central Council for Nursing, Midwifery and Health Visiting (2001b) *The PREP handbook.* UKCC, London

United Kingdom Central Council for Nursing, Midwifery and Health Visiting (2001c) *Professional self-regulation and clinical governance.* UKCC, London

United Kingdom Central Council for Nursing, Midwifery and Health Visiting (2001d) *News.* UKCC, London: last updated August 2001, accessed 15.8.01 http://www.ukcc.org.uk/news

Section 2

In this section you will begin to see how the three strands of legal, ethical and professional introduced in *Section 1* are plaited together and applied to your practice. The topic areas to be covered are:

> ❖ Responsibility.
> ❖ Accountability.
> ❖ Negligence.

Responsibility

Some definitions will be looked at first and then you will be asked to identify aspects of your everyday life for which you are responsible. As soon as you commence training as a nurse you begin to be responsible for a variety of things and when you go out into clinical practice, even for the first time this list grows. Discussion of some of these will help you to understand the implications of accepting responsibility.

As a registered nurse you are responsible for students you teach and supervise. If you are a student's clinical assessor your role encompasses more than just responsibility, you are accountable for that student, as will be discussed later in this section.

> Activity: Brainstorm what the word responsibility means to you.

Compare your answer to a selection of definitions provided by other nursing students:

- ❖ Liable, dependable.
- ❖ An obligation, duty.
- ❖ Being trusted.
- ❖ Completion of tasks.
- ❖ Willingness to do something.
- ❖ Something given to you when you've shown you can do it /earned it.
- ❖ Being in charge of a given situation.
- ❖ Taking charge of expectations.
- ❖ Standing by what you believe in.
- ❖ Being aware/concerned for others.

Some students used phrases like 'being accountable for your actions'; 'making intelligent, educated judgments' and 'facing the consequences'. You will see as you progress through *Section 2* that these phrases are more akin to a definition of accountability, so if you wrote similar definitions keep them for later as there is a link between responsibility and accountability.

Pearson and Vaughan (1991) define responsibility as, 'accepting a task or duty you have been given'.

Thus, there are two components to responsibility: one being asked or charged to do something and the other accepting this task willingly.

Activity: Make a list of things you are responsible for in your everyday life.

It is impossible to give a definitive list as we are all individuals, but your list may contain aspects such as caring for children, exercising the dog, feeding the cat, taxing and insuring the car, doing the shopping, laundry and paying household bills.

Activity: Select one task from your list and identify what this
responsibility involves and why.

Again, it is impossible to provide a specific answer because it
depends on what you choose.

However, there may be some very sound reasons for undertaking that responsibility. The list below provides some of these.

- the law says you must
- fear of punishment
- it is the right thing to do — morally/ethically/honestly
- it is what is expected by others or society in general
- it may be because you always have done it and are
  conditioned into doing it without thinking any further.

Responsibility is personal and derives from being a citizen and
human being.

As a nurse if you have agreed to undertake a task there is an
expectation that you will do it to the best of your ability, safely and
correctly. Safety is the required level of ability of students in the
common foundation part of the pre-registration course. This requires
you to have:

1. **Knowledge** of what the task
    is and why you are doing it.
2. The **skill** to perform the task.
3. An appropriate **attitude** to the
    patient/client.

This is likely to include the ability
to communicate effectively and
demonstrate that you value the
patient's/client's individuality, dignity
and privacy. The triangle here
demonstrates the link between these
prerequisites.

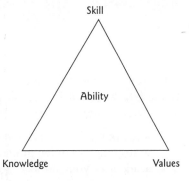

According to Bergman (1981), ability is one of the preconditions necessary to become firstly responsible and ultimately
accountable. You will return to Bergman's work later in this section.

Student nurses' responsibilities

From the first day of any pre-registration course, students take on responsibilities. Attitudes to one's own learning and that of other students are very important. The student is immediately responsible for; attending lectures, punctuality, respecting others' desire and need to learn, being committed to and involved in the course, being self-directed and motivated. Other areas of responsibility require you to act upon advice/guidance/feedback from academic staff and begin to develop your portfolio of learning. These may seem very obvious and are not exclusive to nursing students.

Nursing students are also responsible for their health and are required to have the relevant immunisations and vaccinations prior to commencing clinical practice. Another important area includes the need for a police check to ensure that the student is a suitable person to be caring for others and the student has a responsibility to provide any relevant information relating to this. There are links here again with professional issues because, as you discovered earlier, the NMC must ensure that the public is protected.

Activity: In addition to the above what do you think student nurses will be responsible for on their first clinical placement?

The list below identifies many of these responsibilities and is linked to the UKCC's (2001a) learning outcomes and the range of UKCC and NMC documents currently in use. The responsibilites are to:

- work under supervision of a qualified nurse
- respond to advice/guidance given by supervisors
- identify yourself as a student
- participate in care delivery
- refuse to participate in procedures for which you have not been fully prepared
- respect the wishes of patients/clients
- foster appropriate, non-judgemental attitudes
- behave in a professional, appropriate manner

- provide care which is evidence-based and of a high standard
- maintain written and verbal patient confidentiality
- ensure that all written and computerised records are both accurate and countersigned
- ensure that your personal appearance upholds the professional standard of nursing
- share responsibility for the environment of care
- report complaints to a relevant person
- report untoward incidents to an appropriate person.

Activity: You may wish to make the links with the *Code of professional conduct* by identifying, for each responsibility listed, which clause of the code is most pertinent. You will also find that other UKCC booklets refer to some of these in more detail.

It can be seen that nurses have responsibilities to patients, relatives, colleagues, society and themselves (Rumbold, 1999).

Responsibility is often linked to roles: different roles have different responsibilities. Compare the responsibilities of the first placement student with a more senior student, or a student with a registered nurse. Adult branch nurses may have different roles from child, mental health or learning disabilities nurses. If you are a clinical supervisor your role will be expanded to encompass this with additional responsibilities. Heath (1995: 244) summarises these points quite well stating that, 'these responsibilities must be commensurate with the level of education and training of a nurse or student'.

Implications of responsibility

If you refer back to some of the reasons why you undertake the personal responsibilities you listed at the start of this section, the implications of failing to take them show similarities. For example, as a nurse, if your practice contravenes the Health and Safety at Work Act (1974) there may be **legal** implications for you and/or your employer.

If you fail to practice to the standard set by any of the NMC guidelines a complaint may be made. In the first instance as a student this may be to your clinical supervisor or clinical manager who may reprimand you and advise you how to improve your practice. Continuing failure to practice appropriately could result in failure to achieve the learning outcomes required by the UKCC. This could mean that a student would be unable to continue training.

If there is serious inappropriate behaviour, such as theft or patient abuse, immediate withdrawal from training is likely, in addition to possible legal consequences.

Registered nurses who fail to practise or behave **professionally** may be disciplined by the NMC, as you have discovered in *Section 1*.

Most nurses, at some time during their careers, experience occasions when their conscience is troubled by aspects of their work or that of others. This can result in feelings of discomfort, anxiety and concern about continuing as a nurse. For students with little experience this can be quite distressing and should be voiced so that they can be supported through such experiences and learn from them. Support is available from clinical supervisors; managers; clinical link/liaison teachers; personal tutors and other academic staff as well as other students and nursing colleagues. Even when qualified, the nurse will often find such support is required. These are **ethical** issues so once again the three strands which form the basis of this text are woven together.

It can be seen that student nurses become responsible very early on and need to understand what this means and entails. The UKCC's (1998a) *Guide for students of nursing and midwifery* emphasises this important aspect both to protect the public and enhance the profession of nursing.

Accountability

By the end of this part you should be able to define accountability and give examples of the origins of accountability with reference to a variety of literature. You should be able to differentiate it from responsibility and identify the prerequisites of accountability. To whom you are accountable will be determined and some aspects of accountability in practice will be discussed. The consequences of accountability in relation to standards of care will be outlined.

The NMC (2002) *Code of professional conduct* clearly states in Clauses 1.3, 2.2 that, 'as a registered nurse or midwife, you are personally accountable for your practice' while the previous document, *Guidelines for professional practice* (UKCC, 1996: 8) added, 'accountability is an integral part of professional practice'. What does this mean?

Earlier in this section some students indicated phrases more indicative of accountability than responsibility. Examples included: making judgements; being called to account and justifying what you did; being answerable for and facing the consequences of one's actions.

Many people confuse responsibility and accountability, maybe because there are links between them. Marks-Moran (1996) says that responsibility and accountability are closely connected but are not the same and should not be used synonymously, while Tschudin (1996) reinforces this indicating that although the two do overlap and depend on each other, they are not the same.

Bergman (1981) illustrates the links in her model of the preconditions leading to accountability below:

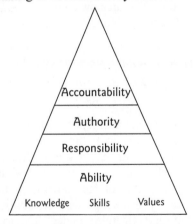

You will remember that the lower levels of this triangle were used when discussing responsibility earlier (*p. 31*).

The **authority** arises from the position you are given and accept, which in turn allows you the power to make decisions. Decision-making involves making judgements in a wide variety of circumstances. This suggests that you also need to be autonomous, being given the freedom to make those choices. Walsh (1997) includes this in saying that to be accountable is to have responsibility both to self and others while having the authority to act autonomously.

Young (1991) links the degree of accountability to the degree of authority and says that nurses cannot be accountable without authority. Lewis and Batey (1982) similarly suggest that authority is needed to carry out actions for which you can be held accountable.

Where does the authority come from?

As a student in the foundation part of a nursing programme, authority is given to you by the training body, in partnership with the university where you are studying. When you undertake clinical practice it is your clinical supervisor who gives you the authority to participate in care delivery. At first this is under supervision but, as you move into the branch, authority increases in line with your more senior status. Both responsibility and authority are linked to this developing role where you may be judged as capable of giving some aspects of care unaided. Once qualified the authority is given by the NMC, as part of being on the register, and your employer within the job description which applies to your post. You are now considered to be **accountable**.
Young (1995: 17) states that:

> *Accountability is not a word that is used within a legal context but is important professionally... legally it is a concept closely related to that of duty of care and negligence.*

Professionally, you may delegate responsibility to someone else but not accountability; this remains with the person doing the delegation who must ensure that whoever they ask to undertake a task/duty is able to perform that task correctly. The individual asked to perform the task must say if they do not feel capable as the NMC (2002: Clauses 6.1–5) outline, 'you must possess the skills, knowledge and abilities for lawful, safe and effective practice'. This forms an important part of the relationship between a student nurse and clinical supervisor.

> *No one else can answer for you and it is no defence to say that you were acting on someone else's orders.*

UKCC, 1996

Student nurses are never professionally accountable in the same way as registered nurses and the UKCC (1998a) states that it is the registered nurse with whom you are working who is professionally accountable for the consequences of your actions and omissions. However, as a student you can be called to account by the law or the university who is training you.

To summarise, professional responsibility and accountability are not the same, the key differences being:

- responsibility has to be accepted
- you can be inexperienced but still have responsibilities, whereas accountability comes with experience
- responsibility can be delegated but accountability cannot
- someone must give you authority before you can be accountable
- accountability requires you to make autonomous decisions
- you must be prepared to answer for your actions to be accountable.

> Activity: List who you think the registered nurse is accountable to.

Figure 2.1 provides a summary (adapted from Dimond, 2002: p.5) demonstrating that the law is an integral part of nurses' accountability.

The student nurse who undertakes any aspect of care which the supervisor is unaware of ('going off on a frolic of her own!') will have put herself into a position of being accountable. The student could be accountable to all in *Figure 2.1* except the NMC. Can you recall from *Section 1* why this is an exception?

Student nurse duties can include what you say, write or do. In the case of what you say, you are accountable because no one else puts words in your mouth. What you write requires countersigning by a registered practitioner so, although you are responsible, the registered nurse is accountable. *Section 3B* will explore the standards required in relation to written communication.

The same situation arises in relation to what you do, as it should be under supervision or with the knowledge of the supervisor who considers you to be competent. This would be in agreement with your own perception as the NMC (2002: Clause 6.3) indicates, you must seek help from a competent practitioner until you have acquired the requisite knowledge, ability and skill.

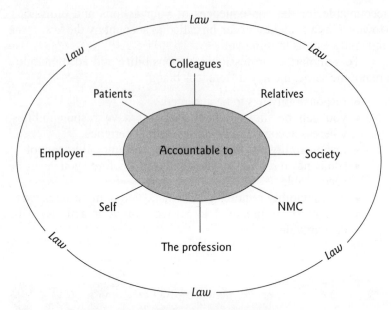

Figure 2.1: Spider diagram of nurses' accountability

Two expressions are used in relation to accountability — acts of commission and acts of omission — these incidentally are nothing to do with Acts of Parliament. If you provide care, which you know is of a poor or incorrect standard, for example, dragging a patient up the bed, this is an **act of commission** for which you could be held accountable. Although you may have repositioned the patient and made him more comfortable the manner in which you did it was unacceptable. You should also consider things not done which should have been. These are called **acts of omission**.

Both qualified nurses and students can commit acts of commission and acts of omission.

Activity: Can you think of three acts of omission?

Answer:

- ❖ You may have thought of not completing some type of chart, such as an observation or fluid balance chart although you did perform the task.
- ❖ Failing to follow a procedure or policy correctly, for example, not informing a detained mental health patient of their rights under the Mental Health Act (1983).
- ❖ Not passing on information to the rest of the multidisciplinary team despite the patient giving you permission.
- ❖ Not explaining a child's care to a parent.

Acts of omission are often not intentional but the consequences for the patient could be serious as you will see later in this section on negligence, as the student is accountable under common law.

Nurses are expected to uphold the good standing and reputation of the profession irrespective of their status. Professional accountability incorporates legal, moral and ethical aspects and sets a very high standard for nurses.

The implications of accountability may appear to be similar to those identified at the end of the responsibility section (look back if you have forgotten, *pp. 33–34*). Identify the variety of sanctions that could be imposed by the following and explain why:

NMC   Employer   Society   Colleague   Self

It depends on the severity of the sanction but anything which means you cannot continue as a nurse can be catastrophic. Being removed from the register as a result of a criminal conviction or being found guilty of professional misconduct may end the career of a registered nurse. Being dismissed from the course as a student will prevent you from getting on the register in the first place. Sometimes an employer may dismiss you but you may still be able to work elsewhere as a nurse provided that you remain on the professional register. The views of colleagues or your own disgust or self-hatred can be very hard to deal with and may result in your choosing to leave nursing. Moral and ethical implications can be just as strong as legal or professional sanctions, the latter are just imposed by someone else.

To help you apply all this to practice try this activity.

Activity: Read the following fictional scenarios and decide who you think is responsible and/or accountable.

Use Bergman's prerequisites of accountability mentioned earlier and think about whether the student should be able to undertake the duty.

Note anything else you think is significant or could help you make a decision, for example, identify the Clauses of the *Code of professional conduct* and ethical principles which you think may apply. In doing this activity you will once again be drawing together the threads which run throughout this text.

Scenario 1

Mary wishes to have a shower and as you helped her to have a bath two days ago you feel confident that you are able to do this unsupervised. Mary finishes her shower and asks you to pass her the towel. Unfortunately she drops it on the shower floor where it rapidly becomes too wet to use. 'Don't worry, Mary', you say, 'I'll just pop and get another one, I won't be a minute'. On your return you find Mary is unconscious on the floor half out of the shower. She appears to have tried to step out of the shower to put on her dressing gown.

Scenario 2

You have a very good clinical supervisor who has worked with you all morning. Together you have just finished washing an elderly, mentally ill and dependent gentleman. This is a new experience as most of the patients you have met have been self-caring. The gentleman is now comfortably sitting in a chair so your supervisor says, 'Just comb his hair and do his mouth and I'll start the drug round, join me when you've finished'. She rapidly disappears before you have time to reply. You are aware that this client has a history of swallowing difficulties and is an epileptic.

To conclude, Tingle (1990) states that however accountability is defined, it is important to remember that the courts are the final venue for the resolution of disputes in medicine and nursing.

Negligence

The first two parts of this section have focused on professional issues in relation to nursing practice but this final part will look at one legal implication of poor practice to complete the picture, that of negligence.

Activity: Look up the word negligence in a dictionary from a legal perspective.

Answer: The variety of definitions you may have discovered could include a failure to exercise proper care and attention.

Heath (1995: 254) says that, 'any nurse who does not meet accepted standards of practice or who performs duties in a careless fashion runs the risk of being negligent'.

Activity: Can you recall what type of 'wrong' negligence is?

Answer: It is a civil action which originates from common law.

You will be looking at some actual cases (which have been simplified in this book) to determine the components that have to be proved by the claimant if they are to win the case. Reference will be made to professional documents which help to set standards of care and may be used in legal situations.

Activity: To whom does the word 'claimant' refer?

Answer: This is the person who has suffered some harm or loss (McHale *et al*, 1998).

The defendant is either the individual practitioner who is alleged to have caused the harm or the organisation which employs the practitioner. Check back to the legal part of *Section 1* (*p. 6*) if you've forgotten how this is referred to in most literature. In most cases which involve nurses it is their employer who is taken to court as the purpose of negligence is to sue for compensation and very few nurses would be able to pay if the case is proven.

The reason the employer is identified in negligence cases is because they take responsibility for the actions of the employee. This is known as the principle of vicarious liability and the employer must be insured against employees' actions which may cause harm to colleagues and/or patients. Vicarious liability only applies if the employee is working within their normal employment which is explained in the contract of employment and job description (Fletcher and Buka, 1999). The basis of proof is one of a balance of probabilities, which means that there must be a greater than fifty per cent chance of the act causing or contributing to harm (Moody, 2001) and that there was a failure to follow a reasonable standard of care.

Harm is one of the four aspects which claimants must prove. These aspects or components of negligence are illustrated in *Figure 2.2*.

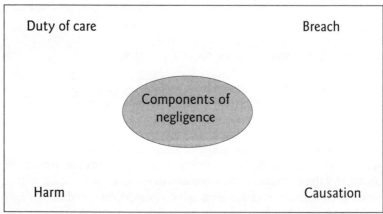

Figure 2.2: Components of negligence

Duty of care

One of the main roles of a nurse is to care for patients and it is not usually very difficult for the claimant to prove this if the nurse was on duty and working within the guidelines determined by the employer and profession. This is clear from the NMC (2002: Clause 1.4). If the nurse is off duty the situation may be different because legally the nurse does not have a duty to intervene, although professionally, the NMC (2002: Clause 8.5) states that in an emergency a nurse has a professional duty to provide care. If this occurs in, for example, a road accident, 'then she takes on a legal duty to care for the person properly' (UKCC, 1996: 11) and hence a duty of care would exist and the expectations would be greater than that of the average passer by. Therefore, by accepting a task, a duty of care exists and there is an expectation that the care provided will be of a reasonable standard.

Breach of duty of care

Rules and regulations are written to both guide and protect and they contribute to the standard of care that a patient may expect from a nurse in a given situation. You should now be aware of the origin of many of these rules and regulations which form the professional guidelines, such as the *Code of professional conduct* (NMC, 2002).

There are also policies and procedures produced by employers which help determine what standard is set, for example, manual handling or infection control policies. You may be able to recall statutory laws which relate to these, such as Health and Safety at Work Act (1974), Public Health (Control of Diseases) Act (1984). It is the practitioner's responsibility to find out what the standard is, ignorance is no defence in law.

Despite all this guidance, rules may be broken, either deliberately, when someone takes a 'short cut' perhaps, or unintentionally. In negligence terms, this is a breach in a duty of care. The claimant has to prove what standard of care was required and how it was breached. To assist in this the question of what is reasonable needs to be answered.

> Activity: What does the word reasonable imply?
>
> Answer: It means doing what is proper, sensible, rational, something that is justifiable.

The case which set the standard or precedence for reasonableness is known as the Bolam test (*Bolam* v. *Friern Barnet* [1957] 2 All ER 118 in Dimond, 1995: 30; UKCC, 1996: 11).

Bolam was a patient who was given electro-convulsive therapy (ECT) and the practice at that time (1950s) did not usually involve giving a muscle relaxant or anaesthetic. As a result, the plaintiff suffered fractures and sued the health authority. Bolam failed to obtain compensation because at the time this was the accepted procedure and many other doctors in that field followed the same practice. In other words, this was the accepted standard of the day and the actions of the defendant were reasonable under those circumstances.

In the case of a nurse then, the test of reasonableness says that the standard is not that of the highest skilled nurse but of the ordinary skilled nurse who is practising that skill competently (Staunch *et al*, 1998: 290).

There have been other precedence cases such as *Whitehouse* v. *Jordan* ([1981] 1 All ER 267 in Dimond, 1995; Staunch *et al*, 1998: 293–295) which have added to this question of what is reasonable. In *Whitehouse* v. *Jordan*, although there had been an error of judgement on the part of the obstetrician, he had been acting in a reasonable way.

These two cases highlight the fact that there may be differing bodies of opinion or sound reasons for not adhering to the accepted principles without being found negligent.

Was harm caused?

For a negligence case to be considered by a court the claimant must have been harmed in some way, unlike professional misconduct cases which do not have this requirement. The harm must also be the sort which is compensatable in law. This is often of a physical nature as it is easier to prove but psychological or financial harm, such as loss or damage to property, may also be compensatable. In addition, the harm must be reasonably foreseeable due to the duty of care being breached.

For example, if a nurse assesses and records that a patient has a high risk of developing pressure sores and does not implement actions to prevent them it is probable that the patient will develop such sores. The failure to act is the breach of duty of care and it is well known that patients at high risk are much more likely to acquire pressure sores.

This example also illustrates the fourth component of negligence, ie. **causation**. The cause of the harm needs to be directly linked to the breach in the duty of care.

Consider the case of a seriously ill child who has meningitis. A doctor prescribes antibiotics but the dose he gives is ten times the normal dose. The child becomes deaf. Was the doctor negligent and was the harm caused because of the doctor's actions? It appears at first that this is a clear case of negligence as the doctor had a duty of care which he breached by giving an incorrect drug dose and the child suffered harm as a result. But was the deafness caused on balance of probabilities by the overdose of antibiotics? Meningitis is an infection which can result in deafness so it is not possible to conclude that it was the drug overdose alone that caused the harm, so negligence cannot be proven (*Kay* v. *Ayrshire and Arran Health Board* [1987] 2 All ER 417 in Dimond, 2002: 46).

Sometimes the claimant does not know that any harm has been caused until many years after an event as the many cases related to asbestosis have shown. Now the claimant has three years from the realisation of harm to sue for negligence. For example, a female patient has a sterilisation as a means of contraception and is told it will be impossible to conceive. She becomes pregnant several years later and it is at that time she realises the harm and can begin a claim for negligence.

Activity: Read the scenarios presented below which are based on real negligence cases to test your understanding. Use the four components that have to be proved by the claimant and decide for each:

❖ Who was negligent?
❖ How was their duty of care breached? Were the defendant's actions reasonable?
❖ What harm was caused? Was it foreseeable?
❖ Was causation directly a result of the breach of duty of care?

You may think that more than one person was negligent in some of the scenarios; identify them and explain how they could also have been negligent.

Scenario 1

A premature baby required oxygen therapy in the neonatal unit. This required careful and continuous monitoring of oxygen concentrations in the baby's blood via a probe inserted into a blood vessel. A junior doctor inserted the probe into a vein instead of an artery. A senior doctor also made the same mistake. As a result, inaccurate oxygen levels were recorded. The baby was given too much oxygen by a nurse as a result of this. The baby suffered permanent damage to the retina of the eye and blindness.

Wilsher v. *Essex Health Authority* [1986] 3 All ER 801 (Dimond, 2002: 45, 56–57) and *Wilsher* v. *Essex AHA* [1987] QB 730, CA (Staunch *et al*, 1998: 287).

Scenario 2

A patient presented at the hospital with symptoms of a chest complaint. The possible diagnosis included tuberculosis (TB); Hodgkin's disease, a potentially fatal disease if not treated early enough, and two other conditions. The doctor decided to perform an invasive procedure and biopsy to help determine which condition the woman had rather than wait for sputum results which would confirm TB.

The procedure carried a risk of damage to a nerve affecting the vocal chords.

The patient sued because this did occur. The results of the sputum test later showed a diagnosis of TB.

Maynard v. *West Midlands Regional Health Authority* [1984] 1 WLR 634 (Dimond, 2002: 40–41; and Staunch *et al*, 1998: 290–291).

Although many of the cases referred to concern doctors, nurses can learn from the decisions made in such cases.

In the two scenarios you have just read the decisions made are summarised below.

Scenario 1

1. All three practitioners owed a duty of care to the baby and the baby did suffer harm.
2. The nurse did not breach her duty of care because she administered oxygen based on the blood levels and could not have known that the doctors had incorrectly positioned the probe. Neither could the nurse be expected to recognise developing retinal damage as this is beyond her role and ability. She acted in a reasonable way.

3. The junior doctor did not breach his duty of care because, although he inserted the probe incorrectly, he had asked his superior to check it. The junior doctor's actions were reasonable in asking for confirmation. The Bolam test applied.
4. The senior doctor was found negligent because he breached his duty of care by failing to notice that the probe was in the wrong place. This resulted in harm to the baby which was foreseeable.

This case went to the House of Lords who held that the claimant had not proved that the excess oxygen had caused the blindness and they ordered a re-trial because of the issue of causation (Dimond, 2002: 57).

Scenario 2

The doctor had a duty of care but there were different expert medical opinions as to whether this was breached. Some experts stated that they would have gone ahead with the biopsy without waiting for the sputum results because of the severity of one possible diagnosis. Others would have waited rather than expose the patient to a procedure which carried risks.

Eventually, after appeal to the House of Lords, the original decision of negligence was overturned based on equally acceptable differences of opinion, both of which were reasonable in the circumstances. The House of Lords stated that:

> *It was not sufficient to establish negligence for the claimant (sic) to show that there was a body of competent opinion that considered the decision was wrong, if there was also a body of equally competent professional opinion that supported the decision as having been reasonable in the circumstances.*

Dimond, 1994

The burden of proof lay with the claimant who could not establish that the actions were unreasonable based on a balance of probabilities.

From these scenarios you can see that there is much for the claimant to prove and opinions of other practitioners in that field are sought to support the case. The question of what is reasonable is very important along with the aspect of causation. Many cases first found on behalf of the claimant go to appeal and even to the House of Lords where the initial decision may be overturned. This is a very lengthy procedure, fraught with problems for the claimant who may choose to settle out of court.

It is important to emphasise that for the nurse, documentary evidence can play a crucial role in recalling events many years after the alleged negligence case has occurred.

To summarise — implications for the nurse

As a student practising under the supervision of a registered nurse it should be almost impossible to be sued for negligence. However, if a student knowingly colludes with a registered nurse and does not follow recommended guidelines, policies and procedures they can find themselves answering a negligence claim in the civil court.

It is important that you keep up-to-date with current evidence and research which is made widely available in nursing literature and know what are the accepted standards of care.

You must ensure that your records are current, accurate and relevant. In *Section 3B* you will look at written communication further.

The registered nurse should be aware of areas which have arisen in both professional discipline and negligence cases and be extra vigilant in these areas of practice.

References

Bergman R (1981) Accountability — definition and dimension. *Int Nurs Rev* **28**(2): 53–9

Dimond B (1994) Standard setting and litigation. *Br J Nurs* **3**(5): 235–8

Dimond B (1995) *Legal Aspects of Nursing*. 2nd edn. Prentice Hall, London

Dimond B (2002) *Legal Aspects of Nursing*. 3rd edn. Longman, Harlow

Fletcher L, Buka P (1999) *A Legal Framework for Caring*. Macmillan, Basingstoke

Heath HMB, ed. (1995) *Potter's and Perry's Foundations in Nursing Theory and Practice*. Mosby, London: unit 3, chapters 12, 13

Lewis F, Batey M (1982) Clarifying autonomy and accountability in nursing services. Cited in: Jones M (1996) *Accountability in Practice*. Quay Books, Mark Allen Publishing Ltd, Salisbury, Wiltshire

Marks-Moran D (1996) cited in Tschudin V, ed. (1996) *Ethics: Nurses and Patients*. Baillière Tindall, London

McHale J, Tingle J, Peysner J (1998) *Law and Nursing*. Butterworth-Heinemann, Oxford

Moody M (2001) Why nurses end up in court. *Nurs Times* **97**(8): 24–6

Nursing and Midwifery Council (2002) *Code of professional conduct*. NMC, London

Pearson A,Vaughan B (1991) *Nursing Models for Practice*. Butterworth-Heinemann, London

Rumbold G (1999) *Ethics in Nursing Practice*. 3rd edn. Baillière Tindall, London

Staunch M, Wheat K, Tingle J (1998) *Sourcebook on Medical Law*. Cavendish, London

Tingle J (1990) A duty of care. *Nurs Times* **86**(30): 60–1

United Kingdom Central Council for Nursing, Midwifery and Health Visiting (1992a) *Code of professional conduct*. 3rd edn. UKCC, London

United Kingdom Central Council for Nursing, Midwifery and Health Visiting (1996) *Guidelines for professional practice*. UKCC, London

United Kingdom Central Council for Nursing, Midwifery and Health Visiting (1998a) *Guide for students of nursing and midwifery*. UKCC, London

United Kingdom Central Council for Nursing, Midwifery and Health Visiting (1998b) *Guidelines for records and record keeping*. UKCC, London

United Kingdom Central Council for Nursing, Midwifery and Health Visiting (1998c) *Guidelines for mental health and learning disabilities nursing*. UKCC, London

Walsh M, ed. (1997) *Watson's Clinical Nursing & Related Sciences*. 5th edn. Baillière Tindall, London

Young AP (1991) *Law and Professional Conduct in Nursing*. Scutari, London

Young AP (1995) The Legal Dimension. In: Tingle J, Cribb A, eds. *Nursing Law and Ethics*. Blackwell Science, Oxford

Additional reading

Castledine G (1999) Professional misconduct case studies. Nurse who undertook a procedure outside her competence. *Br J Nurs* **8**(21): 1419

Castledine G (2000) Professional misconduct case studies. Patient who was left unaccompanied in the bath. *Br J Nurs* **9**(6): 325

Gardner JH (1992) Where the buck stops. *Nursing* **15**(3): 14–16

Kendrick K (1995) Accountability in practice: Part 1. *Prof Nurse* **10**(7): 1–4

Rowe JP (2000) Accountability: a fundamental component of nursing practice. *Br J Nurs* **9**(9): 549–52

Section 3

Introduction

This section is very broadly entitled 'communication' as nurses spend a lot of time doing this. The title was chosen because it reflected a section in the UKCC's (1996) *Guidelines for professional practice* and, to adhere to the *Code of professional conduct* (NMC, 2002) good communication skills are vital. The subsequent content and division has followed the pattern outlined in this document. When nurses communicate it is by word of mouth, non-verbal (body language) and written means. Even these activities have legal, ethical and professional implications, as the two parts of Section 3 will demonstrate. *Section 3A* will focus on the issues of truthfulness/truth-telling, choice, consent, autonomy and advocacy while *Section 3B* will view the many aspects of written communication.

You may find some of the material in this section more complex than in previous sections. This is because many of the issues being tackled are in themselves very complicated, so do not despair. As difficult issues are addressed in this section you will find a higher proportion of references and further suggested reading.

Section 3A

To start with you need to think about a couple of situations to set the scene.

> **Activity:** List situations when you might be asked to disclose personal information.

Your list may contain items such as: bank or building society, child's school, doctor's surgery, reception or offices which deal with tax, benefits or housing issues.

In addition, there are many times when people may be called to give personal information about their health — accident and emergency departments, outpatients' departments and specialised clinics related to sexual or mental health issues.

> **Activity:** Think about the sort of environment that would encourage you to disclose personal information? Also, what characteristics would you like the listener to demonstrate?

You would probably like an environment that is quiet, private and comfortable and where you would not be overheard. You will want the listener to be somebody you can trust, who is relaxed and attentive. When this person explains something, you would want them to talk in a language you understood. You would also not want to feel pressurised into revealing more than you wished. More sophisticated thoughts might include, what are 'they' going to do with this information?

This is fairly standard, common sense thinking with only a little borrowed from psychology. Is this thinking translated into action in a healthcare setting?

Rights, responsibilities/duties

For many years there has been discussion over 'patients' rights'. Different patients' charters have been written by the Department of Health to indicate the standards patients/clients could expect when receiving health care. More recently, the Human Rights Act (1998) has set out a series of expectations anyone can expect from life. Rights are often used as a means for individuals to get their own way. However, for every 'right' a person has there is also a 'duty' or 'responsibility'. The above examples will have identified some of the duties of the person receiving the information.

Dimond (1999) discusses the links between these two complementary factors in parts of her book. In the introduction (p.xiii) to her book, Dimond states that a patient has a **legal right** to:

1. Health care (but not absolute).
2. A reasonable standard of care.
3. Give consent.
4. Access health records.
5. Confidentiality.
6. Complain and have complaints dealt with speedily and effectively.

In addition, Thompson *et al* (2000: 141) argue three more:

the **ethical right** — to know
                — to have privacy
                — to treatment.

To counterbalance rights, Dimond (1999) highlights that patients/ clients also have responsibilities or duties.

The duties include giving as much information as they can to medical/nursing staff about their medical history, relevant family history and any treatment/medication.

If the patient is then given instructions on treatment and care they have a responsibility to carry these instructions out, or else a duty to report to the staff that this has not happened.

If a patient has an appointment for consultation or treatment then they need to give advance notice of inability to attend. If they are subsequently admitted to hospital then it is important that they co-operate as much as possible with the staff and comply with any rules, eg. no smoking policy. There would also be an expectation that they are considerate to other patients and staff. If there is any cause for a complaint then they should report this as soon as possible.

To return to the lists above, not only do patients have responsibilities and duties corresponding to their rights, but nurses also have responsibilities and duties towards patients and clients.

> Activity: Try to think of the duties/responsibilities a nurse has in response to patients' rights listed above.

Patients'/clients' rights	Nurses' duties/responsibilities
A right to health care	Nurses have a legal and professional duty to care for patients/clients (UKCC, 1996)
A right to a reasonable standard of care	Nurses must adhere to the standards in the *Code of professional conduct* (NMC, 2002) and other UKCC documents
A right to consent	Nurses must gain consent prior to any nursing procedure (NMC, 2002)
A right of access to health records	Nurses must abide by the Data Protection Act 1998 and UKCC, 1998b (see *Part B*)
A right to confidentiality	Nurses must adhere to Clause 5 (NMC, 2002) and UKCC documents
A right to complain	Nurses need to apply the policies/procedures of the trust organisation in which they work
A right to know (legal right)	Nurses need to give information honestly and truthfully (NMC, 2002)
A right to privacy	Nurses need to respect Clause 2 (NMC, 2002) and UKCC (1999)
A right to treatment	Nurses have a duty to provide treatment whether active or palliative (Thompson *et al*, 2000)

All this may seem as if the nurse has no rights, but that is not the case. However, that issue will not be addressed here. Another series of points that need to be mentioned here are outlined by Thompson *et al* (2000: 144):

- having rights does not mean that one is bound to exercise them
- having rights does not mean that their exercise is unlimited
- patients' negative rights are in general stronger than positive ones — that is the right to refuse treatment. If a treatment is subsequently given against the patient's/client's will, it is technically criminal assault.

This leads the discussion to the key right of consent, which will now be explored.

Consent

A lot has been written on this subject which covers legal, ethical and professional boundaries. This subject will now be explored from the nursing perspective although it is fully acknowledged that nurses are not the sole custodians of consent. Issues will be raised which may have branch specific variations so alternative methods of handling the differences will be discussed.

At the beginning of this section it was identified that when communicating there were a range of things that you would ideally want in place before divulging personal information. Hopefully this is how you might conduct an assessment interview with a patient/ client on admission, or during your time with them. This is the time when you get to know about them and start to determine what they expect from their time in your care. You may determine how anxious they are, how much, if anything, they want to know about what is wrong with them and how ready they are to discuss implications of their disease process. All this has implications for the nurse when they ask a patient for their consent for a nursing procedure.

Activity: Look at the following two definitions of consent and compare and contrast them. Decide which definition you would prefer to be applied to you if you were in hospital — and why.

1. A voluntary, uncoerced decision made by a sufficiently competent or autonomous person, on the basis of adequate information or deliberation, to accept rather than reject some proposed course of action that will affect him or her (Gillon, 1985).

OR

2. An individual is entitled to sufficient knowledge about his or her condition and proposed treatment with explanations of alternative treatments to be able to make a rational decision regarding treatment choice and, subsequently, be capable of empowering physicians and health care workers to pursue a particular treatment offer (Brykczyńska, 1989).

Both definitions contain elements which are expected before a decision is made by the patient/client. Competence/rationality is required by the person giving consent and information needs to be given to them which will help them make a choice. The definitions differ on the outcome. Gillon (1985) states that after all the input, the person will accept rather than reject what is offered. Brykczyńska (1989) on the other hand, talks of alternatives and the patient/client taking the initiative to empower those who will provide the treatment/care.

There will be some people reading this who, if they were the patient/client, would want to find out all about the treatment/care on offer but at the end of the day would trust the healthcare professionals to do the best for them. Others would want to know about the choices on offer, but would want to make their own choice. There will be another group who would wish to be 'left in the dark' about what could go wrong or finer details of the proposed care and again, trust the healthcare professionals.

When a nurse is assessing a patient/client there needs to be careful exploration of the amount of information the patient/client wants to hear so that when the time comes for a decision there are fewer things for the patient/client to worry about. Once the nurse has established the level of information required this detail must be clearly recorded in the nursing records. Another facet that the nurse must be aware of is the level of understanding that the patient/client has and the ability to make a rational decision. Nurses are not expected to do a deep psychological analysis but to be aware of that person's competence to grasp any information given so that the approach taken is at an appropriate level. Factors that could hinder the understanding of information could include deafness, the disease process itself, distractions or difficulty in understanding English.

All this is leading to the point as to when consent is required for the nurse to undertake a particular procedure. The Department of Health (DoH, 2001) has produced a leaflet giving twelve points on consent that needs to be read in conjunction with the *Code of professional conduct* (NMC, 2002: Clause 3). Many of the points discussed in these leaflets will now be explored.

> Activity: Read these two documents now to help you understand what follows.

Why is consent needed?

If a nurse approaches a patient and, without any positive indication on the part of the patient/client, carries out the procedure (however well intentioned) then the patient has the right to pursue legal action (Dimond, 1999; Fletcher and Buka, 1999; Tingle and Cribb, 1995; Power, 1997; Wicker, 1991).

This could be trespass, which could include:

- a civil or criminal action for battery — if touched without permission
- a civil action for assault — fear of being touched.

There are times when consent would not be required.

Life-threatening emergency

This could be if a person has a cardiac arrest. Unless the patient/client had expressly stated that he/she did not want cardiopulmonary resuscitation (CPR) then it would be expected that CPR would be carried out if considered medically appropriate.

When a patient is sectioned under a relevant Section of the Mental Health Act (1983)

Medication can be given without consent. See later discussions.

Where public health is at risk — Public Health (Control of Disease) Act 1984

A patient/client may need to be isolated in a single room in hospital because of an infectious disease — consent would be requested but could be overridden for the health needs of the majority.

How can a patient/client give consent?

> ❖ Expressly/explicitly
> ❖ Tacitly/implicitly
> ❖ Hypothetically

> Activity: Think of examples of these different ways of giving consent.

Expressly/explicitly

As the words imply, this type of consent gives a clear indication of agreement or approval. It can be in a written form or verbally by the patient/client saying, 'Yes' to getting out of a chair to be weighed. A simple nod of the head is also acceptable. It is fairly unusual for nursing consent to be gained in a written format, but nurses often have to deal with 'consent forms' that have been completed by medical staff. Nurses need to be aware of the importance of consent forms and these will be discussed further in *Section3B*.

> Activity: Find and read the consent forms which are currently being used in your own area of practice. Compare them with other examples you may be able to find in the literature, eg. Dimond (1999: 41) and Brazier (1992: 76).

Tacitly/implicitly

It could be argued that everyone in a hospital setting has given his or her permission for any procedure. This would be taking implied consent too far (McHale *et al*, 1998). Much more commonly this type of consent can be seen in non-verbal communication. If you approach a patient/client with a syringe, and they are expecting to have an injection then an arm or leg may be exposed for you to administer the injection. No words may have been spoken but the gesture is tacitly saying that you have that individual's consent.

Hypothetically

This type of consent is given in a, 'if such and such happens then...' context. There are two key types of hypothetical consent that a nurse will rarely gain, but may well have to act upon. These are when a person has an organ donor card or has written an 'advance directive' or 'living will'.

Who gains consent?

According to the DoH (2001), and the NMC's (2002) edition of the *Code of professional conduct* (see *Appendix 1*), the best person to seek consent is the person carrying out the treatment. There may be times when this can be delegated, but only if that person is both capable and specially trained.

When is consent needed?

Nurses are involved in many types of treatment and care where consent is required. Any procedure requires some form of consent and this is normally by agreement through nodding the head, saying yes or offering the appropriate part of the body. Therefore, express/ explicit, tacit/implied types of consent are used.

Consent is also required for discharge from hospital or for any kind of transfers within or to somewhere outside a hospital. Again, this is not normally in writing but a record of the decision must be made.

Depending on the type of ward environment and trust protocols, written consent is required for some drug treatments such as chemotherapy and treatments under the Mental Health Act 1983. The latter requires agreement by a 'second opinion doctor'.

Consent is required for surgical procedures and invasive tests (including some blood tests) but these are not normally the nurse's responsibility.

For all types of consent there must be validity.

What makes consent valid?

There are several factors which have to be adhered to. Consent must be:

* Voluntary — the individual must not be under sedation or manipulated into a situation of agreement.
* Informed — the nature of the treatment, the risks involved, subsequent consequences and any alternatives must be given truthfully. A very interesting study was undertaken by Taplin (1994) about patients' perceptions of consent. It is very worrying to read, showing low levels of understanding by patients/clients.
* To cover the act to be performed — if a patient/client has requested assistance with a bath, this does not mean that the nurse can also wash the patient's hair, cut his toe nails and trim his beard.
* From a legally competent source — this is a tricky one in that Fletcher *et al* (1995) state that there are no fixed criteria by which to assess competence. There are laws and specific instructions, which need to be adhered to, of who may give consent. See also Tingle and Cribb (1995: 102–104).

Who can give consent?

Adults

No adult can give consent on behalf of another adult, even if the recipient of care is incompetent. However, there may be situations when the carers/relatives/friends are asked for their suggestions as to how the individual would normally react, but could not sign a consent form. Consent needs to be given by the person concerned.

> Activity: The above is the legal point of view, what could be the ethical and professional issues here?

Minors

A parent, or someone to whom parental responsibility has been given, can give consent for treatment to a child. The law specifies the definition of consent and its boundaries.

According to the Family Law Reform Act (1969) for medical, surgical and dental purposes a child can give consent to treatment when aged sixteen. A later Act of Parliament, the Children Act (1989) states that the wishes and feelings of the child should be ascertained and considered in the light of his/her age and understanding. This is obviously going to vary according to the child's mental age and experience.

> Activity: Can you think of any situations when there might be a clash of wills over consent relating to a 'minor'?

Much has been written on this subject, so to avoid repetition why not read some case studies and examples that can be found in the reading list at the end of this section.

Vulnerable clients

Included in this category could be those who are elderly, mentally incapacitated and mentally ill. Some people may be mentally incapacitated for a short time due to sedation or unconsciousness. When looking in the literature, please note that some books also put children into this client group.

There are many people who fall into this category of vulnerable clients. Overall, the principle which must be applied is that the best interests of the patient/client must be paramount. 'Best interests' goes wider than best medical interests and should include factors such as the individuality and wishes of the patient/client when they were competent (eg. advance directive), their current wishes, their general well-being and their spiritual and religious welfare (DoH, 2001).

Trying to provide care in the best interests of the patient/client is not always easy to give accurately. For example, relatives of older people, although they cannot formally give consent to treatment, can influence the care that is given but may not always reflect the patient's wishes at that time. This could be because many older people are tired of living and watching close friends die. When younger they may have undergone treatment to stay alive, but now they are ready to die. This does not imply that they would want to end their lives, just not to prolong them. In this instance, non-intervention would be their choice if able to give their consent.

Activity: Using the legal perspective that has been outlined, think about the ethical and professional problems you might encounter in your area of practice. The literature at the end of this section may help you.

With clients who are mentally incapacitated with learning disabilities from any cause, then relatives, carers and friends may be able to give an indication of the client's wishes. However, there are some specific and clear guidelines in the UKCC's (1998c: 7–8) booklet relating to consent and its validity.

The basis for valid consent is that it must be voluntary, informed, cover the act performed and be from a legally competent source but, in addition, the UKCC (1998c) emphasises that a nurse must:

- act in the best interests of the patient/client
- ensure that the process of establishing consent is rigorous, transparent and demonstrates clear professional accountability
- accurately record all discussions and decisions.

Once again, there are many supplementary sources of information with examples and case studies which can be found in the reading list at the end of the section.

When dealing with mental health patients/clients all the factors listed above apply, but there are other legal aspects a nurse must consider relating to the Mental Health Act 1983.

The Mental Health Act 1983 identifies two groups of patients/clients:

1. Voluntary patients/clients are those who have asked for treatment and are sometimes called 'informal' clients.

2. Detained/sectioned patients/clients who have complex mental health problems and who may have no insight into their condition, are 'detained' for their own or the public's safety.

Following the 'Bournewood case' there is now another group recognised by the House of Lords. This involves patients/clients who are incapable of giving consent to admission to hospital and have **not** been detained under the Mental Health Act 1983. The staff have a duty of care to act in the patients'/clients' best interests under common law powers (DoH, HSC/122, 1998).

Consent should always be sought from mentally ill patients/ clients but there are some differences. A voluntary or informal patient/client can refuse to have treatment when asked for consent. This refusal must be respected unless there has been such a deterioration in that person's condition that they then fall in to the second category and have to be detained under an appropriate section of the Mental Health Act 1983. Common law powers to treat in the patients'/clients' best interests must be observed. Then, as Gunn (1995) describes, there are legal requirements of mental health nurses when dealing with consent issues. Someone who is detained under one of several sections in the Mental Health Act 1983 may be prescribed medication for his/her mental health disorder. The medication may be given by any means, initially and thereafter, for three months. A reassessment is made and treatment continued or amended for a subsequent three months. Correct forms and strict records must be kept of the client's detention status and ability to consent.

This section has looked at a variety of factors relating to the concept of consent. Most of the issues discussed have related to the legal aspects and the impact this has on the nurse working as a professional. You may have noticed that there is no law on consent, but the issues arise from other areas of law.

Here is a summary of the laws involved:

Branch specific	Legal source
General principles	Trespass, assault, battery, negligence, common law principles
Child branch	Family Law Reform Act, Children Act
Mental health	Mental Health Act, Mental Health Act Code of Practice
Learning disabilities	Children Act (if under 16), Mental Health Act, if appropriate

It is now very important to fulfil the earlier promise of considering the ethical and professional issues related to consent. The concepts to be considered will be those of truth-telling or truthfulness, choice, autonomy and advocacy.

> Activity: Look back in *Section 1* and check the name of the person who outlined five ethical principles. How do his principles relate to this section?

One aspect of consent that has been mentioned but needs re-emphasising is that of **informed consent** — as Thompson *et al* (2000) stressed, the right to know. Any patient or client from any of the groups discussed above needs to have information about the choice that they have to make. The choice may be to accept one or other option or refuse the treatment on offer.

For the patient/client to be able to do this the information needs to be given truthfully but in a way that enables understanding, and at a rate that is acceptable to the individual. That is why the importance of individual assessment was highlighted at the beginning of this section. If the patient/client is to have autonomy, the choice that is given must not be one of 'take it or leave it' or 'Hobson's choice' variety. There needs to be a genuine choice and, as stated earlier in this section under validity, the consequences of each option need to be given.

The nurse's duty of care includes the duty to inform — see details on the Bolam test with regards to negligence in *Section 2* (*p. 44*). This means that any breach is actionable, but only if harm can be proved. This is contrasted with trespass where harm does **not** have to be proved.

Truth-telling/truthfulness

From the earlier activity you should have been able to identify Thiroux (2001) as the author of this principle (and the other one of autonomy). Telling the truth is a value which is usually encouraged in early childhood. Thiroux (2001) endorses this and says it is one of the hallmarks of true communication.

Rumbold (1999: 15) suggests this activity:

> Activity: Ask yourself whether you agree or disagree with the following statements:
>
> ❖ To tell the truth is right.
> ❖ One should tell the truth on all occasions.
> ❖ There are occasions when to tell a lie is justified.

You probably said that you agree with the first statement, but that you could argue for and against the other two.

The truth comes in many forms and sometimes the truth may not be suitable as it is too blunt and sounds uncaring for the individual to cope with. Does that mean a lie has to be told, or will you be 'economical' with the truth?

Think of some of the problems which could follow a lie. You will have to remember what you said for a start and then warn everyone else of what you have said so that they could maintain the story. At a later date if you are somehow confronted with the lie, you may lose all trust and credibility.

Economy with the truth can also pose problems. You could easily be confronted with the fuller version of the truth and have to explain your actions, even if this may have been done to minimise the harm (non-maleficence) to the patient/client. Whichever route you take there will be pitfalls.

The NMC (2002, Clause 3.1) says that:

> *Information should be accurate truthful and presented in such a way as to make it easily understood.*

By being sensitive to a patient's needs, there may be rare occasions when a person's condition might lead you to be selective (although never untruthful) about the information you give. How can a nurse tell the truth about a procedure? Consider this scenario:

Nurse: Hello Mr Grant, I've come with your suppositories.
Mr Grant: What are they for?

Nurse:	You said you were very constipated. They help the bowel to work.
Mr Grant:	How are you going to put them in?
Nurse:	If you get on to your bed, turn over on to your left side with your bottom near to the edge, then I will insert them having lubricated them first.
Mr Grant:	Will it hurt?
Nurse:	It may feel a bit uncomfortable, so you need to try to relax.
Mr Grant:	How quick do they work?
Nurse:	You'll get some sensation to want to have your bowels open quite quickly, but you need to try to hold on for about twenty minutes for them to work properly.

On the face of it there is nothing wrong with the exchange between the nurse and Mr Grant, however:

- did he have a choice?
- is a choice necessary?
- did the nurse outline any other consequences apart from success?

The possible need for immediate access to a toilet was not mentioned and the controversial 'truth' that 'if I insert these badly I could actually rupture your rectum' was not mentioned either.

What would you consider to be adequate as consent to this procedure?

This example may be considered simple, but it does illustrate some of the points previously mentioned. Sometimes nurses have to face up to problems of truth-telling which are not of their making. The one which is often quoted is that of discussing diagnosis/prognosis with the relatives without the patient's knowledge or vice versa. Examples of this scenario are illustrated in the appropriate section of the reading list.

An area where telling the truth in action can be difficult is if a patient/client refuses vital medication. There has been a lot of debate over this issue and court cases have followed when patients have been given medication in a disguised form. The UKCC (2001f) has issued strict guidelines if a patient/client is unable to give informed consent and the medication is in their best interests. Disguised medication must never be used for the healthcare team's convenience. In effect, the nurses are not telling the truth in their actions, as they administer drugs disguised in food or drink, but it may be seen as ethically the best course of action as the principle of least harm is being applied.

Truth-telling is only the first part of giving information as, after this information has been given, then the patient/client has a choice. This is where autonomy comes in.

Autonomy

Activity: Find a definition of autonomy.

Thiroux (2001) argues that:

> *... people, being individuals with individual differences, must have their own ways and means of being moral... to follow the dictates of their own intelligence and conscience as much as possible.*

To do this they have to have an opportunity to choose. They also need sufficient information to make the choice (Fletcher and Buka, 1999). The options put before a patient/client should be in their best interests, and also set in the context of the 'common good' of the patients/clients in that part of the wider health service (Thompson *et al*, 2000).

When people in the healthcare setting have a choice they tend to follow one of four routes when confronted with needing to give consent to a procedure. These are:

Choice 1. A patient/client can agree with the nurse and submit to the procedure.

Choice 2. The patient/client may ask a lot of questions — to which the nurse must reply truthfully or equally truthfully, acknowledge his/her limitations (NMC, 2002: Clauses 3 and 6) before a decision can be made.

Choice 3. The patient/client may first agree to the procedure and then later refuse.

Choice 4. The patient can refuse to have the procedure — for a variety of reasons.

These are four ways of expressing personal freedom or autonomy.

At the beginning of *Section 3A* we looked at two definitions of consent. Gillon (1985) assumed that, 'the patient would accept rather than reject some course of action that will affect him or her'. This is the assumption most of us (if truly honest) would make when asking for a patient's/client's consent. How do we handle the situation when a person refuses outright, as in the medication example above? The easy bit is to record 'drug refused' on the medication record.

Activity: What else needs to be considered?

The temptation, when someone refuses something that is offered and considered to be the best course of action, is to try to persuade him/her to change his or her mind (see Fletcher *et al*, 1995: chapter 4; Thompson *et al*, 2000: chapter 7). This is described in some books as 'paternalism' — the idea that, 'we know best, so you must follow our instructions' (Smith, 1994). This does not allow for the patient's/client's individual freedom. Having argued this, some people may say that to have a choice is very confusing, and that in fact the healthcare professionals do know best (Tingle and Cribb, 1995: chapter 6 part B). It is one thing to stand in a supermarket and try to decide which brand of baked beans to buy but quite another to make a decision about surgery or drug therapy.

The next temptation which the authors have regrettably seen in their experience, is that the patient/client receives verbal and non-verbal messages from the staff. These messages could include:

- intense pressure to conform
- remarks which indicate the staff's displeasure
- ostracism
- reduced levels of care.

Unfortunately, what has happened is that the staff do not know how to deal with the situation of rejection, they take it personally and are responding accordingly.

If we believe it is a person's right to choose, as highlighted in many of the previously used texts, then we have to accept the person's right to refuse as well. The care we give to that individual may change to accommodate the different care required, but the standard must be as high (NMC, 2002: Clauses 1.4, 6.5).

Autonomy is not always possible. Many people do not have the capacity to choose. It is very important to create opportunities for autonomy and also to respect the autonomy an individual can cope with. Clearly an infant, an unconscious patient and some people with learning disabilities and mental health problems will not be able to make an autonomous choice (Rumbold, 1999).

When it is necessary to create autonomy in certain circumstances this can be done by gently putting the situation back into the patient's/client's hands and giving them time to think about their decision. Often nurses are in such a hurry that there is little time for the patient/client to deliberate and so they make the choice they think the nurse would like. Not everybody behaves in this way. There may be occasions when you might see your colleagues behaving in a less than helpful way towards a patient/client who is exercising their autonomy as they want. Such a situation might require you to undertake an additional role — that of an advocate.

Advocacy

An advocate is one who pleads on behalf of another. Advocacy, according to Teasdale (1998), is about power: influencing those who have power for those without.

> Activity: In your everyday life, when might you act as an advocate for another?

Your answer may include speaking to a teacher on behalf of your child, acting as a go-between for friends who have quarrelled or signing a petition for or against something.

Advocacy is also a role which is used in the courts and that is why it is sometimes considered to be 'high powered'. It is a role which can be used effectively in the clinical setting to speak on behalf of one, or a group of patients or clients.

One overriding thing which needs to be remembered about advocacy is that the advocate is pleading for the other person and expressing his or her wishes and not the advocate's own.

> **Activity:** Think of different situations when you have or might have to be an advocate for a patient/client.

Your choice of situations will be different according to your area of nursing practice, but there will be similar themes.

❖ The patient/client is unable or unwilling to speak on behalf of him/herself.

❖ You have been one of a group who has campaigned for change, such as a change of time for a procedure.

❖ You defend a patient's or client's decision by speaking to a colleague to explain it.

It is important to add at this point that the British authors who write on advocacy take a much broader view on the subject than do those from North America. Teasdale (1998) gives several examples in his book (chapter 4).

There will be some areas of advocacy which are relatively simple.

❖ A patient/client cannot complete the daily menu sheet and you do it after discussion.

❖ An adult general patient has a visitor come to a hospital ward. Due to a nursing procedure it is inconvenient for the visitor to see the patient for some time. The nurse acts as advocate for the patient when asking the visitor to return in an hour's time. It is a request that may not be acceptable and the patient cannot ask for himself.

❖ Another example could be where a qualified children's nurse in the accident and emergency department discovers that the drug dose prescribed for a three-year-old is twice the dose it should be. Ethically it would not be in the child's best interest to administer the drug, nor would it value the child's life. Professionally the nurse is accountable for her actions and would have to justify why she would give the large dose if she took that course of action. Legally the nurse could be sued for negligence if harm occurred to the child as a result of the drug overdose. To act as this child's advocate, the nurse needs to return the prescription sheet to the medical officer and ask for the dose to be checked and amended.

Other, more complex areas of advocacy can be seen in the following diagram (*Figure 3A.1*).

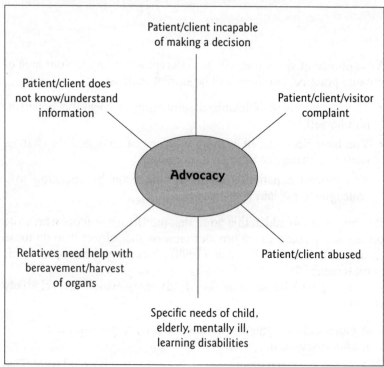

Figure 3A.1: Areas of advocacy

These are all areas where a nurse may get involved. Each of these areas will now be discussed looking at the legal, ethical and professional implications for each.

Patient/client does not know or understand information

This may be after a doctor has spoken to a patient about a procedure. Afterwards the patient asks you what it all meant. You are advised to recall the doctor to answer the patient's questions in a manner s/he can understand. A nurse may only answer questions within his/her level of knowledge (NMC, 2002: Clauses 3, 10, 6), otherwise they may be judged in a court of law as a doctor if a complaint of negligence is made (see *Section 2*).

Patient/client incapable of making a decision

This area of advocacy has been discussed under consent. In all cases the best interests of the patient/client should be paramount.

Patient or visitor complaints

This subject was one of the 'rights' illustrated at the beginning of this section. If a complaint is voiced, you should listen and not comment or act defensively. All trusts have to have a policy for complaints (under the Hospital Complaints Procedure Act 1985; Dimond, 1999) and the nurse acts as an advocate by advising the complainant of the procedure to follow. Sometimes you may have to follow the complaint further if there is need for a report. You would then have to investigate or answer questions to establish whether there was cause for complaint. The outcome may be that you find yourself campaigning on behalf of the patient or relative, because you discover that there is a sound ethical reason for doing so, for example, it is the beneficent thing to do.

Patient or client abused

This is often called whistle-blowing if a member of staff is seen to be abusing a patient or client and misusing the privileged relationship a nurse has (NMC, 2002: Clause 7.1). A recent Act of Parliament, Public Interest Disclosure Act (1998), gives protection to the whistle blower as long as correct procedures have been followed.

Alternatively, you may see a relative abusing a patient/client and have to act as an advocate in a difficult situation. Again, it is important to remember that you are pleading on behalf of someone else and with his or her wishes. The UKCC (1999) outlines types, causes and ways of dealing with all types of abuse of patients or clients. Sometimes abuse is so severe that a criminal case follows. It is also one of the areas considered to be professional misconduct (see *Section 1*).

Specific needs of vulnerable client groups

The elderly, children, those with learning disabilities and mental health problems are vulnerable in different ways. One common denominator is that they are often without power to deal with situations. Sometimes there will be group advocates who may have nothing to do with any healthcare professional. These include NSPCC, Age Concern, Mind and Scope. These groups work on behalf of such client groups and work on common problems although individual needs are also dealt with. According to Gates (1994) these are called collective advocates. Gates also highlights that such client groups may have individuals who are allocated to them to act as specific advocates.

Relatives need help with bereavement or harvesting organs

This situation will obviously depend on where you work. Many relatives need someone to act as an advocate when there has been a death. They may need someone to telephone to find out information which they cannot do in their state of grief.

There are other relatives who find themselves in the position of making a decision about the harvesting of a loved one's organs to donate to another person. At this time, they have a need for someone to act as a go-between so that they understand the process and do not feel too pressurised, particularly while grieving.

This may all sound very positive and a role which nurses would find satisfying. Unfortunately, this is not always so.

Problems of advocacy

There are various problems with advocacy, as it:

- can cause disrupted relationships between colleagues from different disciplines. Teasdale (1998) outlines the many risks an advocate faces in his book
- can lead a nurse to champion one patient but maybe not another, leading to injustice
- can be very time-consuming and therefore be unpopular to the advocate while also making the advocate unpopular as he/she may not be able to share the team's workload equally
- could cause conflict between the nurse's professional role and the interests/wishes of the patient/client.

Recent legislation and advocacy

Human Rights Act (1998)

There are a number of rights which a human being should have which are foundational principles of this Act. Dimond (1999) in her appendix lists these rights. Other chapters in the book outline the continuing effects this law will have.

Public Interest Disclosure Act (1998)

This act has been introduced to protect those who, for whatever reason, have cause to 'whistle blow' in an organisation, provided they follow set protocols. This is obviously a great step forward from ostracism, dismissal and other negative responses individuals have encountered in the past when acting as an advocate.

Table 3A.1 includes questions and actions the advocate may need to consider, producing the differing outcomes listed. For areas/individuals where advocacy may be relevant, see *Figure 3A.1*.

Table 3A.1: Advocacy: Questions, actions and likely outcomes

Question

1. Is it legal?	Yes, OK proceed
	No, eg. Dying patient wants overdose of drugs — cannot proceed
2. Is it ethical?	Yes, OK proceed
	No, eg. Relatives want you to be dishonest on their behalf — cannot proceed
3. Is it professional?	Yes, OK proceed
	No, eg. Patient wants to give you a bribe for preferential treatment — cannot proceed
4. What help is required?	

Actions

Simple advocacy — no risk to advocate

⌘ education   **Outcome**
⌘ explanation   individual acts for him/herself
⌘ encouragement
⌘ empowerment

Intermediate advocacy — some risk to advocate

⌘ speak to another on behalf of an   **Outcome**
   individual   advocate acts for individual who may then
⌘ speak to another on behalf of a group   act for him/herself
⌘ suggest alternatives
⌘ suspend action

Complicated advocacy — high risk to advocate

⌘ communicate widely — whistle to   **Outcome**
   blow?   there may be some results of the action
⌘ challenge system   but this is often at personal cost
⌘ change practice
⌘ count cost — physical, emotional,
   professional

It is important that the advocate reflects on the process whatever level of advocacy is pursued and the consequent outcome.

References

Brazier M (1992) *Medicine Patients and the Law London*. Penguin, London

Brykczyńska G, ed. (1989) *Ethics in Paediatric Nursing*. Chapman & Hall, London

Department of Health (2001) *Health Service Circular HSC 2001/023 Good Practice in Consent*. DoH, London, last updated November 2001, accessed 26.11.01
http://www.doh.gov.uk/hsc200123.htm

Department of Health (1999) *Health Service Circular HSC 1998/122 L* v. *Bournewood Community and Mental Health NHS Trust Decision by the House of Lords in the Appeal*. DoH, London

Dimond B (1999) *Patients' Rights, Responsibilities and the Nurse*. 2nd edn. Quay Books, Mark Allen Publishing Limited, Dinton Salisbury, Wiltshire

Fletcher L, Buka P (1999) *A Legal Framework for Caring*. Macmillan, Basingstoke

Fletcher N, Holt J, Brazier M, Harris J (1995) *Ethics, Law and Nursing*. Manchester University Press, Manchester

Gates B (1994) *Advocacy: A Nurses Guide*. Scutari, London

Gillon R (1985) *Philosophical Medical Ethics*. John Wiley, London

Gunn M (1995) In: Tingle J, Cribb A, eds. (1995) *Nursing Law and Ethics*. Blackwell Science, Oxford: Chapter 8

McHale J, Tingle J, Peysner J (1998) *Law and Nursing*. Butterworth-Heinemann, Oxford

Nursing and Midwifery Council (2002) *Code of professional conduct*. NMC, London

Power KJ (1997) The legal and ethical implications of consent to nursing procedures. *Br J Nurs* **6**(15): 885–8

Rumbold G (1999) *Ethics in Nursing Practice*. 3rd edn. Baillière Tindall, Edinburgh

Smith L (1994) In: Hunt G, ed. *Ethical Issues in Nursing*. Routledge, London

Taplin D (1994) In: Hunt G, ed. *Ethical Issues in Nursing*. Routledge, London: chapter 1

Teasdale K (1998) *Advocacy in Health Care*. Blackwell Science, Oxford

References

Thiroux JP (2001) *Ethics: Theory and Practice.* 7th edn. Prentice Hall, New Jersey

Thompson IE, Melia KM, Boyd KM (2000) *Nursing Ethics.* 4th edn. Churchill Livingstone, Edinburgh

Tingle J, Cribb A (eds) (1995) *Nursing Law and Ethics.* Blackwell Science, Oxford

United Kingdom Central Council of Nursing, Midwifery and Health Visiting (1996) *Guidelines for professional practice.* UKCC, London

United Kingdom Central Council of Nursing, Midwifery and Health Visiting (1998c) *Guidelines for Mental Health and Learning Disabilities Nursing.* UKCC, London: 7–8

United Kingdom Central Council of Nursing, Midwifery and Health Visiting (1999) *Practitioner-client relationships and the prevention of abuse.* UKCC, London

United Kingdom Central Council of Nursing, Midwifery and Health Visiting (2001f) *Register Autumn Number 37.* UKCC, London: 7

Wicker CP (1991) Legal responsibilities of the nurse 3: Assault and Consent. *Surg Nurse* 4(1): 16–17

Additional reading (see specific page references)

Reading related to children's and minors' issues and consent

Chadwick R, Tadd W (1992) *Ethics and Nursing Practice.* Macmillan, Basingstoke: 96–109

Dimond B (1999) *Patients' Rights, Responsibilities and the Nurse.* 2nd edn. Quay Books, Mark Allen Publishing Limited, Dinton, Salisbury, Wiltshire: 38–9

Fletcher L, Buka P (1999) *A Legal Framework for Caring.* Macmillan, Basingstoke: 110

Fletcher N, Holt J, Brazier M, Harris J (1995) *Ethics, Law and Nursing.* Manchester University Press, Manchester: 153

McHale J, Tingle J, Peysner J (1998) *Law and Nursing.* Butterworth-Heinemann, Oxford: 80

Rumbold G (1999) *Ethics in Nursing Practice.* 3rd edn. Baillière Tindall, Edinburgh: 231

Thompson IE, Melia KM, Boyd KM (2000) *Nursing Ethics.* 4th edn. Churchill Livingstone, Edinburgh: 145

Reading related to vulnerable elderly patients/clients

Chadwick R, Tadd W (1992) *Ethics and Nursing Practice.* Macmillan, Basingstoke: 159–61

77

Fletcher L, Buka P (1999) *A Legal Framework for Caring*. Macmillan, Basingstoke: 152

Tingle J, Cribb A, eds. (1995) *Nursing Law and Ethics*. Blackwell Science, Oxford: chapter 9

Reading related to vulnerable mentally ill and incapacitated patients/clients

Fletcher L, Buka P (1999) *A Legal Framework for Caring*. Macmillan, Basingstoke: 122

Fletcher N, Holt J, Brazier M, Harris J (1995) *Ethics, Law and Nursing*. Manchester University Press, Manchester: chapter 10

Health Service Circular (1998) *L* v. *Bournewood Community and Mental Health NHS Trust. Decision by the House of Lords in the appeal (HSC 1998/122)*. NHS Executive, Department of Health, London

Jenkins R (1997) Issues of empowerment for nurses and clients. *Nurs Standard* **11**(46): 44–6

McHale J, Tingle J, Peysner J (1998) *Law and Nursing*. Butterworth-Heinemann, Oxford: 87–98

Rumbold G (1999) *Ethics in Nursing Practice*. 3rd edn. Baillière Tindall, Edinburgh: 236

Truth-telling to patients and relatives

Fletcher N, Holt J, Brazier M, Harris J (1995) *Ethics, Law and Nursing*. Manchester University Press, Manchester: 54

McHale J, Tingle J, Peysner J (1998) *Law and Nursing*. Butterworth-Heinemann, Oxford: 76

Thompson IE, Melia KM, Boyd KM (2000) *Nursing Ethics*. 4th edn. Churchill Livingstone, Edinburgh: chapter 6, 118–119

Autonomy

Dimond B (1999) *Patients' Rights, Responsibilities and the Nurse*. 2nd edn. Quay Books, Mark Allen Publishing Limited, Dinton, Salisbury, Wiltshire: chapter 3

Fletcher N, Holt J, Brazier M, Harris J (1995) *Ethics, Law and Nursing*. Manchester University Press, Manchester: chapter 4

Thompson IE, Melia KM, Boyd KM (2000) *Nursing Ethics*. 4th edn. Churchill Livingstone, Edinburgh: chapter 7

Tingle J, Cribb A, eds. (1995) *Nursing Law and Ethics*. Blackwell Science, Oxford: chapter 6 part B

Section 3B

The final part of this book, *Section 3B*, will look at the vital aspect of written communication. This is an area which is often derided by nurses as, 'just a paper exercise' but this is a key area of nursing practice as highlighted in the UKCC document *Guidelines for records and record keeping* (UKCC, 1998b), and Clause 4.4 in the *Code of professional conduct* (NMC, 2002).

There are numerous legal, ethical and professional issues within written communication. The professional aspects will be looked at first. These will include the types of written material and their importance and the role of the nurse in dealing with written records. Some of the laws which have influenced the professional guidelines will be identified and legal implications for practice will be outlined. Finally, a variety of ethical issues relating to records and record keeping will be discussed as they affect the role of the student and the qualified nurse.

Professional aspects of written communication

The UKCC (1998b: 7) states very clearly in the introduction to their specific guidelines on written communication that:

> *Record keeping is an integral part of nursing, midwifery and health visiting. It is a tool of professional practice and one which should help the care process. It is not separate from this process and it is not an optional extra to be fitted in if circumstances allow.*

Before considering writing anything within the nursing context there are three questions which Castledine (1998) advises you to ask:

- who is going to use or read the information?
- what type of information does the reader require?
- what is the best way of organising and presenting the material?

Now look at how these questions can be answered.

> Activity: Make a list of all the different types of documents that you have to complete in your area of nursing practice.

One of the things you should have on your list is the fact that documents are produced by different means; handwritten and computer generated.

Your list of the types could have been very long indeed, and your frustration at having to do so much paper work may have been clear in your mind at the time!

Nursing records could include:

Care plans:	assessment sheets, plans for specific care, hand written/core care plans, daily summaries of the care given and the reactions to this, evaluations of the care given and subsequent assessments
Charts for:	fluid balance, weight, mood, turning the patient in bed, neurological observations, nutritional intake, temperature, pulse, respiration and blood pressure — to name but a few
Records used by the inter-professional team:	accident/incident forms, discharge letters/ referral letters, consent forms, specific forms for mental health rights, prescription sheets

Some records may well be used by all the above people, and there are also records which are held by the patient/client/parent and are brought to the professional when relevant. These include ante-natal records, children's immunisation records and privately-funded records such as X-rays and second opinions.

> Activity: Who is going to read the documents you have listed?

A vast number of people could, potentially, read any of these documents. Siegler (1987) gives the example of a patient asking how many people would read his documents and was eventually told this was seventy-five. Primarily they will be written for the professional staff who will be using them, eg. nursing, midwifery, medical, professionals allied to medicine (PAMs) — pharmacists, occupational therapists, physiotherapists, speech therapists, radiographers, play specialists, social workers... the list is extensive. It must never be forgotten that the record is about an individual and they have the right to read personal records (see the legal part of this section, *pp. 86–90*). If records are needed for a court case related to any aspect of care then all the personnel involved in that case would be entitled to read relevant parts of the patient's/client's records.

Due to the fact that people from different backgrounds will be reading the records, it is important that they are written in a format that will be understood by all. It is also so much easier and safer to read a record that is in a logical and chronological order.

Whichever record is required, it is important that it is completed correctly. The UKCC (1998b) makes it clear that for records to be effective they must:

- be factual, consistent and accurate
- be written as soon as possible after the event to be current
- be clear and permanent and able to be photocopied
- be unambiguous with any alterations crossed through with the original still being legible. These alterations should be treated as per a cheque, ie. dated, timed and signed
- be accurately dated, timed and signed with the signature printed by the first entry. All records a student completes must be countersigned by a qualified nurse (UKCC, 1998a).

Also, records should not include abbreviations, jargon, meaningless phrases, irrelevant speculation and offensive subjective statements.

Abbreviations: There are many abbreviations which are commonly used in nursing. Many trusts have a list of approved abbreviations for you to use. Any other abbreviation must be written in full and followed by the abbreviation in brackets.

Jargon: Again, in nursing these are commonplace but need to be explained to a patient/client verbally or written in the records.

Meaningless phrases: Usually these are a combination of the above.

Irrelevant speculation: 'This patient will come to a sticky end' is really rather unhelpful.

Offensive subjective statements: No statement in a record should be offensive. A subjective statement is one that is based on your own biased opinion. An objective statement is one where specific facts are included. For example, Mabel has had a home visit today and says she is feeling very tired.

The records should also be written in conjunction with the patient/carer and be written so that they can understand the content. The entries in the records need to be consecutive with clear evidence that care has been planned on the basis of assessment, implemented and subsequently evaluated.

An example of a record that should never have been written is as follows:

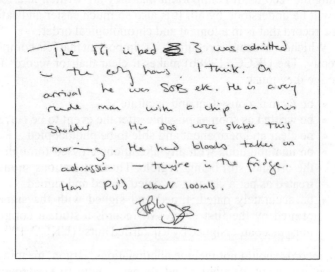

This was all written in pencil apart from the student's signature which was written over white erasing fluid.

Activity: Using the UKCC's checklist above, identify which of the UKCC requirements for effective records have been ignored.

❖ The record is not factual or accurate, eg. 'I think' 'stable'.

❖ It is not dated or timed, therefore, is it current? Was it written as soon after the events as possible?

❖ It is in pencil, anything could be erased and accuracy could be questioned. It is also not photocopiable.

❖ Additions have been made and there are no correcting signatures, nor does a qualified nurse countersign the record. It is unclear who made the record and his/her status.

❖ It contains so many abbreviations, jargon words and meaningless phrases that the record would be difficult for a patient to understand and would be ridiculed in a court of law. (Please see the legal section later as to why the patient needs to understand the record.)

❖ There is a very derogatory sentence in this report that should not be there. What right has the writer of the report to make this judgement on a man who has been admitted in pain following a myocardial infarction?

Discussion points

Think about the abbreviations, eg. SOB — how many ways can you use this abbreviation?

> *Shortness of breath, sat out of bed, American expletive deletive....*

What do you think the 'etc' in the record might mean?

> *It could be that Fred was in pain or that he was suffering all the attendant physical symptoms a person with a 'heart attack' might have.*

PU'd is a terrible abbreviation of passed urine, but is often used.

Points to consider

It is important to write records or complete forms as soon as possible after the event. It is difficult to remember precise details after time has elapsed and you have done a variety of other things in between, even if you know you have got to remember the details.

Another point to remember is that one word could convey a different set of circumstances. For example, both the words 'slipped' and 'fell' could mean an individual was once upright and then horizontal. The means of the change could be related to something external — slipped (on a spilt substance), or internal (due to a change in blood pressure) — fell. The consequences if a court case ensued could be very different.

Simple things can also make such a difference. Consider the following real example. During a court case for compensation for a back injury, one of the documents used for evidence was a card written on by the claimant's GP. The date had been stamped on the card, but a gap had been left above it. The doctor had written in the gap when the claimant had gone to see him with her injuries. Consequently, it looked as if the injury was already there when the alleged accident had occurred.

Hopefully you will not encounter many records written like the above example, but you will see some that come close. Make sure those records are not yours.

A better way of looking at the events reported could be:

Nursing Records

Admission sheet: This would contain all the personal details of the patient and also his baseline observations.

Assessment sheet: This would have looked at all of the patient's needs within a model of nursing.

Care plan: This would identify the way the nurses would be caring for this gentleman. Issues such as his pain, his intake and output and any special pressure relieving instructions should have been included. Such a patient may also be very anxious about himself, his home circumstances and this need must be explored and possibly a referral made for additional support from someone like a social worker.

Additional records

> Activity: Think of other records which might be included in this gentleman's nursing records.
> Items such as prescription sheet, fluid balance chart, pressure sore indicator, record and pain assessment chart could be included.

So far the **writing** of records has been clearly identified as part of the nurse's role.

Activity: What other responsibilities does a nurse have with regard to records and record keeping?

As well as fulfilling the UKCC's guidelines for the writing of records, the nurse's role extends further than completing the writing element already discussed.

The following diagram (*Figure 3B.1*) identifies the many facets to the nurse's role within record keeping.

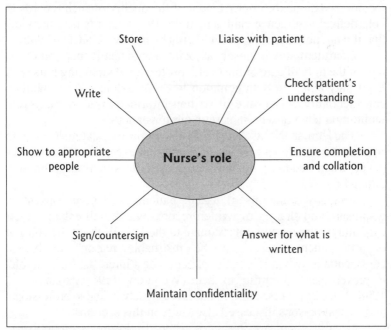

Figure 3B.1: Facets to the nurse's role within record keeping

Legal aspects of written communication

The two main areas of law covered here concern confidentiality of written communication, how and when this may be breached; and the security, protection and access of data.

You have already discovered that numerous people are likely to be involved in healthcare delivery and that, if as many as seventy-five could legitimately need to know something about a patient to provide ongoing care, how can confidentiality ever be maintained? The principles of confidentiality apply to both verbal and written information which may be in a manual and/or computerised form, but the emphasis here will be on written communication.

The law recognises that confidentiality is not absolute (McHale *et al*, 1998: 100) as nursing records may be required by a court as evidence in negligence cases, for example. In addition, the Audit Commission studies records within hospitals and makes recommendations for improvement of the quality of such records to help defend negligence claims (Tingle, 1995). Courts take the view that if it has not been recorded it has not been done (UKCC, 1998b).

Confidentiality is closely associated with negligence and forms part of the duty of care of the health professional including nurses. A legal duty exists in both common law and statute law to maintain confidentiality. Disclosure of written information is only allowed, without patient consent, in certain circumstances.

The Human Rights Act (1998) also imposes a statutory 'right to respect for private and family life' and that exceptions should only occur when required by law under specific situations (Dimond, 2002: 149, 573).

In many situations, if asked, patients will give consent to disclosure and sharing of written records which will enhance their care and treatment without recourse to the law. Without the consent of the patient, there may be justifiable reasons to breach confidentiality when it is in the patient's best interests, for example, to prevent harm occurring to them (Woodrow, 1996; Staunch *et al*, 1998: 221–225). These circumstances are closely linked to professional and ethical reasons discussed elsewhere in this section.

Legally, there are instances when disclosure is compulsory. These include:

❖ **Road Traffic Act 1988** where personal injuries or death occurs, details have to be given to the police .

❖ **Prevention of Terrorism Act 1989** where injuries occur which may be a result of terrorist activities and there is reason to believe that an act has, or is likely to take place.

❖ **Public Health (Control of Disease) Act 1984** requires personal details to be provided to the district medical officer where notifiable diseases such as cholera, smallpox, typhus or food poisoning are suspected.

❖ **Police and Criminal Evidence Act 1984** enables the police to apply for powers via a judge to obtain access to material which is otherwise excluded from this legislation, such as personal records, which are confidential.

Powers of the court

Additionally, a court has the power to order documentary evidence to be provided as well as requiring a healthcare professional to attend as a witness. This is known as a subpoena and it is in the interests of justice. There are some exceptions to these powers, which include issues of national security or legal privilege. Legal privilege does not extend to nurses though.

Public interest

Breach of confidentiality may be justified if it is in the public interest, defined as the interests of an individual, groups of people or society as a whole (UKCC, 1996).

A serious crime may be suspected, for example, rape or child abuse or an individual(s) may be at risk if someone else's health problem is not revealed. Dimond (2002: 56, 57) discusses the problems of public interest as there is very little guidance from the courts apart from the American case of Tarasoff in 1976, and *W* v. *Edgell* [1990] 1 All ER 835 and 1 All ER 855CA. In this latter case, an independent psychiatric report was passed to the Medical Director of W's hospital and a copy was forwarded to the Home Secretary (Brazier, 1992: 54–55). The psychiatrist believed the Home Office should be aware of the client's mental health state. (See also Staunch *et al*, 1998: 254–255; Hendrick, 2000: 99–100.)

This is only a brief summary of some of the legal issues surrounding confidentiality and it is unlikely that any individual nurse will be required to make decisions in relation to them alone. The onus for decision making is more often on the doctor. Other members of the healthcare team, including nurses, may either be the first to be aware of potential conflicts or, be party to the decision to breach confidentiality. Of course, the nurse has to deal with the patient and the consequences of such breaches in a professional and sensitive manner.

There is also legislation which relates to security of, and access to information. The main acts are summarised and you will be asked to think about some of the implications for nurses.

Computer Misuse Act 1990

This broad act aims to combat various forms of deliberate misuse (including 'hacking') which are of public concern. As there is increasing use being made of computerised record systems in all areas of health care, the nurse needs to know the key aspects.

The main offences are:

a. Unauthorised access or intent to access, or to make a computer perform a function, which may enable access to an unauthorised person.
b. Helping someone else commit an offence.
c. Unauthorised modification of contents which may impair computer operation, prevent/hinder access to data or impair the reliability of data.

In other words, this means a deliberate attempt to do something which affects the way that the computer works or change something the computer has recorded so that it affects the information it contains in some way.

If any of these offences are committed and the person is found guilty, a six-month prison sentence and/or fine may be imposed.

This sounds very technical and frightening for those dealing with computerised data, but the purpose is to protect the individual who may have confidential information stored on computer. Nurses must ensure that their practice does not allow anyone without appropriate permission to find out about a patient.

Activity: Find out how this is safeguarded in clinical practice.

Access to Medical Reports Act 1988

This legislation enables clients to access medical reports written for insurance or employment purposes. The client must be told a report is being asked for, give permission and be given the opportunity to see it before it is submitted. If anything is incorrect the client is allowed to amend the report. There are some exceptions to safeguard the client (see McHale *et al*, 1998: 114; Dimond, 2002: 169).

Activity: How may this law apply to you ?

Data Protection Act 1998

This law is an amalgamation of the previous 1984 Data Protection Act and the Access to Health Records Act 1990, most of which it replaces. Like the Computer Misuse Act 1990 it aims to protect individuals from the misuse of personal information (Hendrick, 2000: 106).

The act sets a similar standard to that determined by the UKCC (1998b) guidelines in that, for example, data should be accurate, secure and confidential.

Patients can now apply to see both computerised and hand written information irrespective of how far back the record was made. Earlier legislation restricted manual record access to those written after 1 November, 1991.

Access is requested in writing by the patient to the person who either made the record or, in the case of an institution like a hospital, to the data controller who consults with the professional who made the record. A maximum £50.00 fee can be charged.

Activity: List what **you** think access should include.

Answer: The key points are summarised as:

❖ Inspection.
❖ Explanation.
❖ Copy.
❖ Correction.

Access applies to the patient, a person with written authorisation, a person having responsibility for a child (where the patient is the child), or a person appointed by the court (for incompetent patients).

Access is not absolute as it can be denied or restricted if there is a risk of physical or mental harm to the patient as a result of letting them see their records. There are also restrictions imposed if another person mentioned in the record refuses consent or may be harmed as a result of disclosure (Dimond, 2002: 168).

Activity: Make some notes on the implications of the Data Protection Act for the nurse.
Identify some specific types of situations which you think could arise where access might be denied.

As mentioned earlier, record keeping often comes under scrutiny in negligence cases and patient complaints. Cases and professional literature indicate that, 'most problems occur through failure in basic communication such as poor record keeping and not passing on enough information' (Tingle, 1997). He advises that nurses should develop more reflective practice and keep up-to-date by reading professional literature to help heighten awareness of recurring problems.

Ethical aspects of written communication

Thiroux's (2001) principles relating to ethics were discussed in *Section 1 (p.18)*. These will now be related to written records.

Activity: Think of different ethical aspects which may affect
written records.

Look at the poor example of record keeping illustrated earlier in this
section (*p. 82*).

Value of life

This record did not demonstrate that the nurse valued the patient's
life. He was considered a rude man who had a chip on his shoulder. If
people are anxious they often come across as being rude, and a nurse
needs to remember this and not make unwise judgements. By
labelling a patient, the nurse removes that person's individuality.

Another example of demonstrating this principle is if you
correctly collate documents for certain procedures, eg. prior to surgery;
when mental health rights have to be checked or when social services
discussions have to be processed.

When using patient's/client's records the nurse must maintain
the confidentiality of the contents. For students who are writing case
studies or reflecting on critical incidents, it is important to gain the
consent of the person but still change all the details. By doing this,
you are respecting that individual and recognising that they do not
want private information shared with others.

Goodness or rightness

Records are written and maintained for the continuity of care for an
individual. This is why they always need to be accurate and clear so
that subsequent readers can do the most good for a patient
(beneficence). It would be unethical to show a record (which would
contain personal information) to anyone who asked. There is always
a need to check on the 'need to know' basis. The notion of
confidentiality is based on this principle.

Confidentiality is an ethical issue as well as a legal one. It is
anticipated that records may be seen by a large number of people —
remember Siegler (1987) mentioned earlier? It is vital that a person's
trust in the healthcare team is not destroyed by the breaching of
confidentiality. However, there are some circumstances where a

breach of confidentiality is permitted, but this would need to be following heart-searching and discussions with relevant personnel. The NMC (2002: Clause 5) says that disclosures can only be made with the patient's consent, by order of the court or where you can justify disclosure in the wider public's interest. (This was developed further in the legal aspects.)

(Further discussions on this topic can be found in Fletcher and Buka, 1999; McHale *et al*, 1998: chapter 7; and Dimond, 1999: chapter 4.)

Truth-telling, honesty

This is a highly relevant principle. When writing records it is essential to tell the truth and use the most appropriate words. Look back at the paragraph in this section which refers to the two words, slipped and fell, and the consequences of using the wrong words.

> Activity: Think of another example where similar words could convey different meanings.

In the truth-telling context you need to make sure that the patient understands what is happening or going to happen to them and the possible consequences of the procedure. If the patient is unsure, the UKCC (1996: 18) advises that you tell other members of the health-care team that this is the case, and also act as advocate for the patient by arranging for the appropriate person to come and discuss the situation with them. It is imperative that an honest record is made of any discussion.

By signing or countersigning a document you are saying, 'This is true'. Always read what you are going to sign to make sure that is the case! Don't forget that records may be required in a court of law or for professional misconduct cases.

Justice and fairness

It is in the patient's best interests that they have the option to contribute to the care that they receive and it is only fair that they can have the opportunity to see documents and have these explained to them. This has been discussed in the legal part of this section.

Autonomy, individual freedom

All the examples given above which relate to the patient being involved in their records and the keeping of their records, imply that there is the opportunity for choice. The patient may choose to let the professional staff advise rather than to question. The patient's wishes must be honoured.

You will also need to consider the patient's autonomy when writing records as the patient can challenge what you have written and then you will have to justify your actions, in other words, be accountable. In some circumstances, a patient may personally contribute to the records. For example, completing a fluid balance chart.

Activity: Think of other examples where you give patients the responsibility of an aspect of their records.

Useful facts about records and record keeping

Sometimes it is easier to remember facts if they are put in an unusual format. Using the alphabet, here are some facts to remember about records and record keeping:

A   Nurses are accountable for them.
B   Must be written in black ink.
C   Must be correct, current, comprehensive, chronological, consistent, countersigned and confidential.
D   Should be detailed, dated.
E   Can be used as evidence.
F   Must be written factually.
G   Can be given to patient under the Data Protection Act (1998).
H   Must be honest; and legible when hand written.
I   Must involve patient, carers and significant others.
J   Must be judgement free.

K   Need to be kept for varying periods of time, eg. adults and children.

L   Need to be legible and literate.

M   Should be meaningful and useful to the multi-disciplinary personnel who read them.

N   No-one should make any derogatory comments.

O   Should be objective.

P   Photocopiable.

Q   Should question your practice for improvements when necessary.

R   Demonstrate your rationale for care delivery.

S   Must be signed.

T   Must be timed and dated.

U   Should be unaltered.

V   Should be verifiable and valid.

W   'If it has not been written (recorded) it has not been done'.

X   No mistakes, but if there are, they need to be crossed through and signed.

Y   Always ask, 'Why am I writing this record?' 'Who is going to read it?'

Z   Be zealous for excellence.

QUIZ to consolidate information in this section

1. Why do nurse need to keep records?
2. How should a record be presented? (content and style)
3. Who owns a patient/client record?
4. Make a list of people who have right of access to records.
5. For how long should a record be retained?
6. Why is this time scale set?
7. Name and date some specific laws that relate to health records.
8. Give a summary of each.
9. Under what circumstances can a patient be refused access to his/her own records?
10. Find a definition of confidentiality.
11. Give specific reasons why and when confidentiality may be breached.
12. Using drug administration documents as a focus, identify some of the associated record keeping pitfalls.
13. Which UKCC documents give help and advice to nurses regarding records?
14. Suggest which of Thiroux's ethical principles might relate to records and record keeping, and why.
15. What are the qualified nurse's responsibilities towards a student when the latter is completing a patient's/client's record?

References

Brazier M (1992) *Medicine, Patients and the Law*. Penguin, London

Castledine G (1998) *Writing, documentation and communication for nurses*. Quay Books, Mark Allen Publishing Limited, Dinton, Salisbury, Wiltshire

Computer Misuse Act 1990: chapter 18. Last accessed 27.5.02 http://www.hmso.gov.uk/acts/acts1990

Department of Health (2001) P*atient Confidentiality and Caldicott Guardians — Frequently Asked Questions*. Accessed 17.07.01 http://www.doh.gov.uk/nhsexipu/confiden/faq.htm

Dimond B (1999) *Patients' Rights, Responsibilities and the Nurse.* 2nd edn. Quay Books, Mark Allen Publishing Limited, Dinton, Salisbury, Wiltshire

Dimond B (2002) *Legal Aspects of Nursing.* 3rd edn. Longman, Harlow

Fletcher L, Buka P (1999) *A Legal Framework for Caring.* Macmillan, Basingstoke

Hendrick J (2000) *Law and Ethics in Nursing and Health Care.* Stanley Thornes, Cheltenham

McHale J, Tingle J, Peysner J (1998) *Law and Nursing.* Butterworth-Heinemann, Oxford

Nursing and Midwifery Council (2002) *Code of professional conduct.* NMC, London

Siegler M (1987) cited in: McHale J, Tingle J, Peysner J (1998) *Law and Nursing.* Butterworth-Heinemann, Oxford

Staunch M, Wheat K, Tingle J (1998) *Sourcebook on Medical Law.* Cavendish, London

Thiroux J (2001) *Ethics: Theory and Practice.* 7th edn. Prentice Hall, New Jersey

Tingle J (1995) Why hospital medical record keeping must improve. *Br J Nurs* **4**(17): 982–3

Tingle J (1997) Record Keeping and Negligence. *Br J Nurs* **6**(15) : 889–91

United Kingdom Central Council for Nursing, Midwifery and Health Visiting (1996) *Guidelines for professional practice.* UKCC, London

United Kingdom Central Council for Nursing, Midwifery and Health Visiting (1998a) *Guide for students of nursing and midwifery.* UKCC, London

United Kingdom Central Council for Nursing, Midwifery and Health Visiting (1998b) *Guidelines for records and record keeping.* UKCC, London

Woodrow P (1996) Exploring confidentiality in nursing practice. *Nurs Standard* **10**(32) : 38–42

Conclusion

The following questions may help you to pull together many of the strands that have been identified in this book. They are designed to help you to consider the different issues which have been presented and hopefully will help you see how the legal, ethical and professional issues affect your day-to-day practice as a nurse — student or qualified.

Question 1

Using the *Code of professional conduct* (NMC, 2002), the *Guidelines for records and record keeping* (UKCC, 1998b) and the concept of confidentiality — discuss the legal, ethical and professional issues a student nurse should consider when making an entry in a patient/client record.

Question 2

Consent, truth-telling and autonomy are vital factors to consider when undertaking patient/client care. Discuss the legal, ethical and professional implications of these factors when you are delivering care to a patient/client in your area of practice.

References

Nursing and Midwifery Council (2002) *Code of professional conduct.* NMC, London

United Kingdom Central Council for Nursing, Midwifery and Health Visiting (1998b) *Guidelines for records and record keeping.* UKCC, London

Appendix I

Code of professional conduct

As a registered nurse or midwife, you are personally accountable for your practice. In caring for patients and clients, you must:

- respect the patient or client as an individual
- obtain consent before you give any treatment or care
- protect confidential information
- co-operate with others in the team
- maintain your professional knowledge and competence
- be trustworthy
- act to identify and minimise risk to patients and clients.

These are the shared values of all the United Kingdom health care regulatory bodies.

1 Introduction

1.1   The purpose of the *Code of professional conduct* is to:

- inform the professions of the standard of professional conduct required of them in the exercise of their professional accountability and practice
- inform the public, other professions and employers of the standard of professional conduct that they can expect of a registered practitioner.

1.2   As a registered nurse or midwife, you must:

- protect and support the health of individual patients and clients
- protect and support the health of the wider community
- act in such a way that justifies the trust and confidence the public have in you
- uphold and enhance the good reputation of the professions.

1.3 You are personally accountable for your practice. This means that you are answerable for your actions and omissions, regardless of advice or directions from another professional.

1.4 You have a duty of care to your patients or clients, who are entitled to receive safe and competent care.

1.5 You must adhere to the laws of the country in which you are practising.

2 As a registered nurse or midwife, you must respect the patient or client as an individual

2.1 You must recognise and respect the role of patients and clients as partners in their care and the contribution they can make to it. This involves identifying their preferences regarding care and respecting these within the limits of professional practice, existing legislation, resources and the goals of the therapeutic relationship.

2.2 You are personally accountable for ensuring that you promote and protect the interests and dignity of patient and clients, irrespective of gender, age, race, ability, sexuality, economic status, lifestyle, culture and religious or political beliefs.

2.3 You must, at all times, maintain appropriate professional boundaries in the relationships you have with patients and clients. You must ensure that all aspects of the relationship focus exclusively upon the needs of the patient or client.

2.4 You must promote the interests of patients and clients. This includes helping individuals and groups gain access to health and social care, information and support relevant to their needs.

2.5 You must report to a relevant person or authority, at the earliest possible time, any conscientious objection that may be relevant to your professional practice. You must continue to provide care to the best of your ability until alternative arrangements are implemented.

3   As a registered nurse or midwife, you must obtain consent before you give any treatment or care

3.1   All patients and clients have a right to receive information about their condition. You must be sensitive to their needs and respect the wishes of those who refuse or are unable to receive information about their condition. Information should be accurate, truthful and presented in such a way as to make it easily understood. You may need to seek legal or professional advice, or guidance from your employer, in relation to the giving or withholding of consent.

3.2   You must respect patients' and clients' autonomy — their right to decide whether or not to undergo any health care intervention — even where a refusal may result in harm or death to themselves or a foetus, unless a court of law orders to the contrary.

'This right is protected in law although in circumstances where the health of the foetus would be severely compromised by any refusal to give consent, it would be appropriate to discuss this matter fully with the team, and possibly to seek external advice and guidance' (see clause 4).

3.3   When obtaining valid consent, you must be sure that it is:
- given by a legally competent person
- given voluntarily
- informed.

3.4   You should presume that every patient and client is legally competent unless otherwise assessed by a suitably qualified practitioner. A patient or client who is legally competent can understand and retain treatment information and can use it to make an informed choice.

3.5   Those who are legally competent may give consent in writing, orally or by co-operation. They may also refuse consent. You must ensure that all your discussions and associated decisions relating to obtaining consent are documented in the patient's or client's health care records.

3.6   When patients or clients are no longer legally competent and thus have lost the capacity to consent to or refuse treatment and care, you should try to find out whether they have previously indicated preferences in an advance statement. You must respect any refusal of treatment or care given when they were legally competent, provided that the decision is clearly applicable to the present circumstances and that there is no reason to believe that they have changed their minds. When such a statement is not available, the patients' or clients' wishes, if known, should be taken into account. If these wishes are not known, the criteria for treatment must be that it is in their best interests.

3.7 The principles of obtaining consent apply equally to those people who have a mental illness. Whilst you should be involved in their assessment it will also be necessary to involve relevant people close to them; this may include a psychiatrist. When patients and clients are detained under statutory powers (mental health acts), you must ensure that you know the circumstances and safeguards needed for providing treatment and care without consent.

3.8 In emergencies where treatment is necessary to preserve life, you may provide care without patients' or clients' consent, if they are unable to give it, provided you can demonstrate that you were acting in their best interests.

3.9 No one has the right to give consent on behalf of another competent adult. In relation to obtaining consent for a child, the involvement of those with parental responsibility in the consent procedure is usually necessary, but will depend on the age and understanding of the child. If the child is under the age of 16 in England and Wales, 12 in Scotland and 17 in Northern Ireland, you must be aware of legislation and local protocols relating to consent.

3.10 Usually the individual performing a procedure should be the person to obtain the patient's or client's consent. In certain circumstances, you may seek consent on behalf of colleagues if you have been specially trained for that specific area of practice.

3.11   You must ensure that the use of complementary or alternative therapies is safe and in the interests of patients and clients. This must be discussed with the team as part of the therapeutic process and the patient or client must consent to their use.

4   As a registered nurse or midwife, you must co-operate with others in the team

4.1   The team includes the patient or client, the patient's or client's family, informal carers and health and social care professionals in the National Health Service, independent and voluntary sectors.

4.2   You are expected to work co-operatively within teams and to respect the skills, expertise and contributions of your colleagues. You must treat them fairly and without discrimination.

4.3   You must communicate effectively and share your knowledge, skill and expertise with other members of the team as required for the benefit of patients and clients.

4.4   Health care records are a tool of communication within the team. You must ensure that the health care record for the patient or client is an accurate account of treatment, care planning and delivery. It should be consecutive, written with the involvement of the patient or client wherever practicable and completed as soon as possible after an event has occurred. It should provide clear evidence of the care planned, the decision made, the care delivered and the information shared.

4.5   When working as a member of a team, you remain accountable for your professional conduct, any care you provide and any omission on your part.

4.6   You may be expected to delegate care delivery to others who are not registered nurses or midwives. Such delegation must not compromise existing care but must be directed to meeting the needs and serving the interests of patients and clients. You remain accountable for the appropriateness of the delegation, for ensuring that the person who does the work is able to do it and that adequate supervision or support is provided.

4.7   You have a duty to co-operate with internal and external investigations.

5   As a registered nurse or midwife, you must protect confidential information

5.1   You must treat information about patients and clients as confidential and use it only for the purposes for which it was given. As it is impracticable to obtain consent every time you need to share information with others, you should ensure that patients and clients understand that some information may be made available to other members of the team involved in the delivery of care. You must guard against breaches of confidentiality by protecting information from improper disclosure at all times.

5.2   You should seek patients' and clients' wishes regarding the sharing of information with their family and others. When a patient or client is considered incapable of giving permission, you should consult relevant colleagues.

5.3   If you are required to disclose information outside the team that will have personal consequences for patients or clients, you must obtain their consent. If the patient or client withholds consent, or if consent cannot be obtained for whatever reason, disclosures may be made only where:

- they can be justified in the public interest (usually where disclosure is essential to protect the patient or client or someone else from the risk of significant harm)
- they are required by law or by order of a court.

5.4   Where there is an issue of child protection, you must act at all times in accordance with national and local policies.

6   As a registered nurse or midwife, you must maintain your professional knowledge and competence

6.1   You must keep your knowledge and skills up-to-date throughout your working life. In particular, you should take part regularly in learning activities that develop your competence and performance.

6.2   To practise competently, you must possess the knowledge, skills and abilities required for lawful, safe and effective practice without direct supervision. You must acknowledge the limits of your professional competence and only undertake practice and accept responsibilities for those activities in which you are competent.

6.3   If an aspect of practice is beyond your level of competence or outside your area of registration, you must obtain help and supervision from a competent practitioner until you and your employer consider that you have acquired the requisite knowledge and skill.

6.4   You have a duty to facilitate students of nursing and midwifery and others to develop their competence.

6.5   You have a responsibility to deliver care based on current evidence, best practice and, where applicable, validated research, when it is available.

7   As a registered nurse or midwife, you must be trustworthy

7.1   You must behave in a way that upholds the reputation of the professions. Behaviour that compromises this reputation may call your registration into question even if it is not directly connected to your professional practice.

7.2   You must ensure that your registration status is not used in the promotion of commercial products or services, declare any financial or other interests in relevant organisations providing such goods or services and ensure that your professional judgement is not influenced by any commercial considerations.

7.3   When providing advice regarding any product or service relating to your professional role or area of practice, you must be aware of the risk that, on account of your professional title or qualification, you could be perceived by the client as endorsing the product. You should fully explain the advantages and disadvantages of alternative products so that the patient or client can make an informed choice. Where you recommend a specific product, you must ensure that your advice is based on evidence and is not for your own commercial gain.

7.4   You must refuse any gift, favour or hospitality that might be interpreted, now or in the future, as an attempt to obtain preferential consideration.

7.5   You must neither ask for nor accept loans from patients, clients or their relatives or friends.

8   As a registered nurse or midwife, you must act to identify and minimise the risk to patients and clients

8.1   You must work with other members of the team to promote health care environments that are conducive to safe, therapeutic and ethical practice.

8.2   You must act quickly to protect patients and clients from risk if you have good reason to believe that you or a colleague, from your own or another profession, may not be fit to practise for reasons of conduct, health or competence. You should be aware of the terms of legislation that offer protection for people who raise concerns about health and safety issues.

8.3   Where you cannot remedy circumstances in the environment of care that could jeopardise standards of practice, you must report them to a senior person with sufficient authority to manage them and also, in the case of midwifery, to the supervisor of midwives. This must be supported by a written record.

8.4   When working as a manager, you have a duty toward patients and clients, colleagues, the wider community and the organisation in which you and your colleagues work. When facing professional dilemmas, your first consideration in all activities must be the interests and safety of patients and clients.

8.5   In an emergency, in or outside the work setting, you have a professional duty to provide care. The care provided would be judged against what could reasonably be expected from someone with your knowledge, skills and abilities when placed in those particular circumstances.

Glossary

Accountable   Responsible for something or to someone

Care   To provide help or comfort

Competent   Possessing the skills and abilities required
                           for lawful, safe and effective professional
                           practice without direct supervision

Patient and client   Any individual or group using a health
                           service

Reasonable   The case of Bolam v. Friern Hospital
                           Management Committee (1957) produced
                           the following definition of what is
                           reasonable.
                           'The test is the standard of the ordinary
                           skilled man exercising and professing to
                           have that special skill. A man need not
                           possess the highest expert skill at the risk
                           of being found negligent... it is sufficient
                           if he exercises the skill of an ordinary man
                           exercising that particular art.'
                           This definition is supported and clarified
                           by the case of Bolitho v. City and Hackney
                           Health Authority.

Further information

This *Code of professional conduct* is available on the Nursing and
Midwifery Council's website at http://www.nmc-uk.org. Printed
copies can be obtained by writing to the Publications Department,
Nursing and Midwifery Council, 23 Portland Place, London W1B
1PZ, by fax on 020 74362924 or by e-mail at publications@nmc-uk.org.
A wide range of NMC standards and guidance publications expand upon
and develop many of the professional issues and themes identified in the
Code of professional conduct. All are available on the NMC's
website. A list of current NMC publications is available either on the
website or on request from the Publications Department as above.

Enquiries about the issues addressed in the *Code of professional conduct* should be directed in the first instance to the NMC's professional advice service at the address above, by e-mail at advice@nmc-uk.org, by telephone on 020 7333 6541/6550/6553 or by fax on 020 7333 6538.

The Nursing and Midwifery Council will keep this *Code of professional conduct* under review and any comments, suggestions or requests for further clarification are welcome, both from practitioners and members of the public. These should be addressed to the Director of Policy and Standards, NMC, 23 Portland Place, London W1B 1PZ.

Appendix II

UKCC	NMC
Total of forty practitioners	Total of twelve practitioners
Each country of the UK has seven nurses, two midwives and one health visitor	Each country of the UK has one nurse, one midwife and one health visitor
Twenty lay members appointed by the Secretary of State for Health	Eleven lay members similarly appointed
President Alison Norman (2001–2002)	President Jonathan Asbridge (2002–to date)
Accountable to the Secretary of State for Health and the registered practitioners	Accountable to the Privy Council only

Ref: http://www.ukcc.org.uk/cms/content/Home/Shadow/NMC/Council.asp accessed 14.12.01

Index

A

accountability 34–35, 37, 39
Acts
  ~ Access to Medical Reports Act
    1988 89
  ~ Children Act 1989 62, 64
  ~ Computer Misuse Act 1990 88
  ~ Data Protection Act 1998 89
  ~ Health Act 1999 5
  ~ Health and Safety at Work Act
    1974 33, 43
  ~ Human Rights Act 1998 54, 74,
    86
  ~ Mental Health Act 1983 39, 58,
    60, 63–64
  ~ Nurses Midwives and Health
    Visitors Act 1997 10
  ~ Police and Criminal Evidence Act
    1984 87
  ~ Prevention of Terrorism Act 1989
    87
  ~ Public Health (Control of Disease)
    Act 1984 59, 87
  ~ Public Interest Disclose Act 1998
    73, 75
  ~ Road Traffic Act 1988 86
acts
  ~ of commission 38
  ~ of omission 38
advocacy 70–71, 73, 75
authority 35
autonomy 23, 25, 68–69, 93

B

bill 3
Bolam test 43, 47

C

causation 44
civil liability 1, 6
claimant 6
Code of professional conduct 17, 40, 60
common law 2
compensation 7, 42, 44, 84
Computer Misuse Act 1990 88
conduct
  ~ professional 13
Conduct and Competence Committee
    15
confidentiality 86–89
consent 56–57, 59, 61, 63
  ~ informed 61, 65
  ~ voluntary 61
Coroner's Court 8
crime 6
criminal 1
criminal liability 6

D

Data Protection Act 1998 89
Department of Health 54, 58, 60
disclosure 86
duties 54–55
duty 30
  ~ duty of care 42
  ~ breach of 43

E

ethical principles 40
ethics
  ~ definition 17–18